Delavier's
Core Training
Anatomy

Library of Congress Cataloging-in-Publication Data

Delavier, Frédéric.
  [Des abdos d'enfer. English]
  Delavier's core training anatomy / Frédéric Delavier, Michael
    Gundill.
    p. cm.
  Includes index.
  ISBN-13: 978-1-4504-1399-2 (soft cover)
  ISBN-10: 1-4504-1399-4 (soft cover)
  1. Abdomen--Muscles. 2. Muscle strength. 3. Abdominal exercises.
    I. Gundill, Michael. II. Title.
  QM151.D44813 2011
  613.7'1886--dc22

                                    2011010490

ISBN-10: 1-4504-1399-4 (print)
ISBN-13: 978-1-4504-1399-2 (print)

Copyright © 2010 by Éditions Vigot, 23 rue de l'École de Médecine,
75006 Paris, France

This publication is written and published to provide accurate and
authoritative information relevant to the subject matter presented.
It is published and sold with the understanding that the author
and publisher are not engaged in rendering legal, medical, or other
professional services by reason of their authorship or publication
of this work. If medical or other expert assistance is required, the
services of a competent professional person should be sought.

This book is a revised edition of *Des Abdos D'Enfer*, published in
2010 by Éditions Vigot.

Photography: © All rights reserved.
Illustrations: © All illustrations by Frédéric Delavier.
Modeling and design: Graph'm
Editing: Sophie Lilienfeld

Human Kinetics books are available at special discounts for bulk
purchase. Special editions or book excerpts can also be created
to specification. For details, contact the Special Sales Manager at
Human Kinetics.

Printed in Italy   10 9 8 7 6 5 4 3 2 1

Human Kinetics
Web site: www.HumanKinetics.com

United States: Human Kinetics, P.O. Box 5076
Champaign, IL 61825-5076
phone: 800-747-4457, e-mail: humank@hkusa.com

Canada: Human Kinetics, 475 Devonshire Road Unit 100
Windsor, ON N8Y 2L5
phone: 800-465-7301 (in Canada only), e-mail: info@hkcanada.com

Europe: Human Kinetics, 107 Bradford Road, Stanningley
Leeds LS28 6AT, United Kingdom
phone: +44 (0) 113 255 5665, e-mail: hk@hkeurope.com

Australia: Human Kinetics, 57A Price Avenue
Lower Mitcham, South Australia 5062
phone: 08 8372 0999, e-mail: info@hkaustralia.com

New Zealand: Human Kinetics, P.O. Box 80
Torrens Park, South Australia 5062
phone: 0800 222 062, e-mail: info@hknewzealand.com

E5525

FRÉDÉRIC DELAVIER • MICHAEL GUNDILL

Delavier's Core Training Anatomy

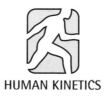

HUMAN KINETICS

Contents

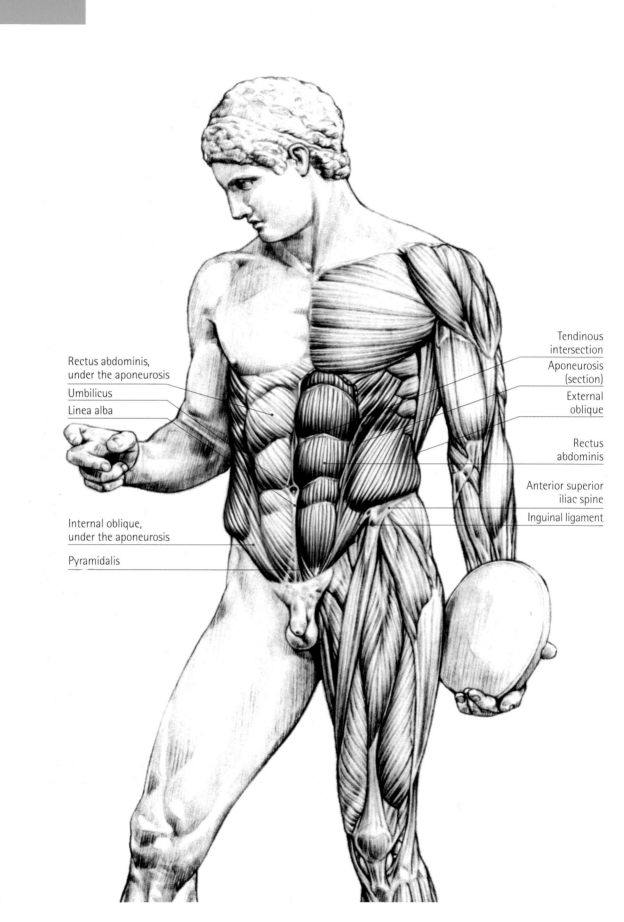

Tendinous
intersection

Aponeurosis
(section)

External
oblique

Rectus
abdominis

Anterior superior
iliac spine

Inguinal ligament

Rectus abdominis,
under the aponeurosis

Umbilicus

Linea alba

Internal oblique,
under the aponeurosis

Pyramidalis

Introduction

When people talk about the abdominal and core muscles, the first thing that comes to mind is appearance: Muscular, well-defined abs are void of fat and synonymous with a flat belly.

However, nature did not intend for these muscles just to look nice: The abdominal and core muscles fulfill vital functions in movement and health. So getting a "six-pack" is not the only reason to exercise these muscles. Beyond your appearance, there are six good reasons to take care of your abdominal and core muscles:

1. Improve athletic performance. The core muscles play a predominant role in all physical activities where you need to run fast or twist your torso, such as golf and tennis.

2. Protect the spinal column. Working with the lumbar muscles, the abdominal muscles provide powerful support to the spine. Conversely, weak abdominal muscles and a prominent belly place the discs in a precarious position, increasing the risk of lumbar degeneration.

3. Relax tense muscles. At night, it is common for the lumbar muscles to stay tense. This means you might wake up feeling tired with a persistent backache. Low back pain in the morning is a sign that your spine did not relax and recuperate during the night. A few minutes of abdominal and core work before bedtime is generally enough to relax your lumbar spine, allowing it to release the pressure it was subjected to during the day.

4. Improve digestive health. Abdominal work facilitates digestion, thereby preventing bloating and constipation.

5. Reduce risk factors for diseases such as type 2 diabetes. This is a disease that occurs as many people age, in large part due to excess belly fat.

6. Maintain cardiovascular health. Exercising the abdominal and core exercises in a circuit is an excellent cardiovascular workout equivalent to running, but without any trauma to the knees and spine.

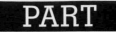
20 Steps to Creating the Perfect Core Workout Program

Creating a workout program for your core will depend on a number of basic theories that you should know. We methodically describe these 20 steps one by one, and they will be the keystone of your personalized program. Learning these 20 steps will help you answer all the questions you might have about creating your workout program.

1 Set your goals.

The very first step in creating your core workout program is to be specific when defining your goals. Are you working out for these reasons?

- To get a six-pack
- To get a slimmer waist
- To maintain your cardiovascular health and fitness
- To increase your athletic performance

Often, your goals may be a combination of several of the items listed. However, if you do not define your goals well, it will be difficult to establish an optimal program. Write down your goals on paper so that you can read them before every workout.

Then, you need to quantify your goals. For example, I want to

- be able to see my abs in 3 months,
- lose 2 inches off my waist in 2 months, and
- double the number of sets I can do in 10 minutes to increase my endurance within 15 days.

The time frame and amount of progress for your goals must be realistic. Keep in mind that no one ever progresses as fast as desired. You might often feel that you have hit a plateau. But with a good program, a true plateau is rare. By quantifying your goals and creating monthly milestones, you will more easily be able to gauge your progress. Each step you achieve will serve as motivation to continue exercising. We provide some typical programs in part 6 of this book. These are basic plans, and you will be able to personalize them using various parameters that we describe next.

2 How many workouts should you do each week?

Your schedule will be the determining factor in answering this question. Unfortunately, your schedule is not always optimal. Just know that if you can work out only once a week, that is still better than not working out at all! You will still make progress. Working out twice weekly is a good minimum. The ideal scenario would probably be three core workouts per week. However, we recommend that you do no more than five workouts per week. Be aware that overtraining slows progress more than undertraining. Only very serious athletes will benefit from daily workouts.

Development

Ideally, you should begin with two workouts per week for a few weeks. When you feel ready, you can move up to three workouts per week. At first, do not go beyond these three weekly workouts. After three months of working out regularly, you could try four workouts per week.

⚠ When you first start working out, you generally have a lot of energy. You feel like working out every day so that you can see results quickly. But this excess enthusiasm can cause you to lose strength rather than gain it—a sign of overtraining! This could make you lose your motivation. Results will not happen instantaneously. If you are careful about how you proceed, you will be able to stick to your program.

3 On which days of the week should you exercise?

You should alternate exercise days with rest days. If this doesn't fit your schedule, do the best you can between what is ideal and what will work for you. Some options:

- **One workout per week:** Choose any day you like.
- **Two workouts per week:** Ideally, your core-specific workouts should be spaced out as much as possible. An example is Monday and Thursday or Tuesday and Friday. In any case, give yourself at least one rest day between two core workouts. The exception is, of course, if you can exercise only on the weekends. Although doing back-to-back workouts is not ideal, you will still have the rest of the week to recover.
- **Three workouts per week:** The ideal configuration is to alternate a day of training with a day of rest. For example, work out on Monday, Wednesday, and Friday. This way your whole weekend is free. It is still possible to do two days of consecutive training (on the weekend, for example) and do the third workout on Wednesday. But you should avoid this as much as possible. The worst program would have you doing core workouts three days in a row. The only way to justify this is if your schedule absolutely requires it.

> ⚠ Knowing how many times per week to work your abdominal and core muscles comes back to asking yourself how many days of rest those muscles require between workouts. Muscle growth occurs only during the rest phase between workouts and not during the actual workout. So it is just as important to know when to rest as it is to know when to exercise. If you are not getting stronger from one workout to the next, it would be wise to allow your muscles more recovery time. If you are not making progress, then you are not getting enough rest.

- **Four workouts per week:** Since there are fewer rest days in this schedule, you will have to work out two days in a row. But if you have a very flexible schedule, you could spread the four workouts over eight days instead of seven days. This way, one day of training will always be followed by one day of rest. The slightly longer training intervals will mean you get an optimal recovery. The only drawback is that your workout days will change from week to week.

4 Should you exercise once or twice per day?

Only champion athletes exercise more than once a day. And they do it only when preparing for a competition! For everyone else, it is better to exercise only once a day and not every day.

If you can work out only once a week because of your schedule, you might eventually want to divide that into two workouts: a session in the morning and one in the evening. You should consider that only after you exercise for a few weeks, though; that program is far from ideal.

The exception is if your goal is to lose inches off of your waist quickly. In this case, you could consider two workouts per day. In fact, doing a circuit of abdominal and core exercises will still burn fat even if the muscle is overworked and not in its optimal shape. Nonetheless, overall fatigue could result. If that happens, you will need to reduce the frequency of your workouts.

5 What time of day should you exercise?

Some people prefer to train in the morning and others in the afternoon or evening. In fact, strength varies depending on the time of day. Some people are stronger in the mornings and weaker in the afternoons. For others, the opposite is true. These fluctuations are caused by the central nervous system and are completely normal. It is rare to find athletes who have consistent strength throughout the day.

> ⚠ Your workout time may be determined by your daily schedule and not by your body. Even if you are not training at the ideal time for your body, the simple rule is that you should always exercise at the same time each day. Your muscles will get used to it, and they will perform their best at that time.

Ideally, you should exercise when your muscles are the strongest. The majority of athletes are strongest around 6 to 7 p.m. This time works out well because it is when many people have the time to exercise.

6 How many sets should you do?

DEFINITION: A set is the number of repetitions of the same exercise that you do until you reach fatigue.

The volume of work is determined by two criteria:
- The number of sets per exercise
- The number of exercises performed

The number of sets is an important factor in muscle development:
- If you do too few sets, the muscles will not be optimally stimulated to grow rapidly.
- If you do too many sets, the muscles will be overworked, which can slow their growth.

Your fitness level determines the number of sets you should do.

As a beginner, do no more than 5 sets.
After 1 month of exercising, do 6 or 7 sets.
After 2 months of exercising, do 8 or 9 sets.
After 3 months of exercising, do 10 sets.

After 3 months, you can decide on your own how many sets you need to do depending on your muscles' needs and their ability to recover. However, you should never do more than 25 sets.

Note: You should always do at least one light set as a warm-up before beginning any core workout (see also page 18). These warm-ups are less intense, and you do not count them in the total number of sets mentioned previously.

⚠ The point is not to do a bunch of easy sets so that you can reach your target number. It is better to work harder with each set and do fewer sets in total than the alternative. If you have no problems going beyond these maximum limits, then it means your muscular contractions are not intense enough. You will acquire this intensity as you train. When you begin, you will not be able to go to the end of your physical limits in a set.

7 Be flexible and adaptable.

The number of sets is the first variable to adjust in the volume of work for your abs and core. It is a smaller adjustment than adding exercises. At first, you have to play around by adding sets rather than increasing the number of exercises. As you become stronger, and when you feel ready, add a set here and there.

The best thing is to let your muscles tell you how many sets you should do. The most obvious indicator is when you start to lose strength abnormally from one set to the next. A sudden loss of strength indicates that you have perhaps done one set too many. You will now know this for your next workout.

Obviously, the number of sets that you can do may fluctuate from one workout to the next. On days when you are feeling great, you might be tempted to add sets. But on days when you are feeling tired, you can reduce the number of sets so that you do not wear yourself out.

You should also keep in mind what you did in your previous workout. If you increased the intensity, weight, or number of sets, expect that your recovery time will be longer. This is why a really good workout is often followed by a poor workout. Because you asked more of your muscles, they need longer to recover. So that your future workouts do not suffer, it is important to have a rest day between workouts.

CONTROVERSY ABOUT SINGLE OR MULTIPLE SETS

There is great controversy about the number of sets you should do for each muscle. Some say that one very intense set per exercise is enough. This is true for certain athletes whose central nervous system has the capacity to give its maximum effort for one intense set. Afterward, they lose a lot of strength and cannot repeat the same effort. In this case, doing a second set of the same exercise would be counterproductive. However, the majority of people don't have this characteristic in their central nervous systems. Scientific research estimates that only 30 percent of athletes have muscles that are better adapted for single sets, while the remaining 70 percent of athletes do better with multiple sets.

That 70 percent group must increase the intensity gradually so that they can give their maximum effort during a workout. They will be frustrated if they do a single set per exercise because their muscles will not be able to express their power completely. They will still have strength left over for another set. In this case, it would be counterproductive to do only one set. These individuals need to do several sets to work a muscle to its maximum.

Multiple sets are also better for the abdominal and core muscles since the goal is to strengthen the muscles and shed the layer of fat covering them.

A single set will in no way help eliminate fat that is resistant to a diet. Only a serious amount of core work has a chance at eliminating the fat.

8 How many exercises should you do for each muscle?

During each workout, you have two choices:

1. Do only a single abdominal or core exercise.
2. Perform two or three different exercises

The choice here is not so difficult if you know the advantages and disadvantages of each strategy. Your fitness level will also prove to be a determining factor.

Single Exercises: A Good Beginning Strategy

When you begin, you should choose a single exercise (one that is best suited for you—we explain how to choose it later on). Later, you can add another exercise to increase the intensity. You can increase the number of exercises as you get stronger.

Advantages of a Single Exercise

Fortunately, most people like a routine and are happy doing their favorite exercises. This attitude is preferable if you are a beginner because repeating an exercise will improve your technique in performing that exercise.

In fact, the abdominal and core muscles cannot give their best effort during a new exercise. They require an initiation phase (called motor learning) so that they can mobilize their full power during an exercise. This is why you make rapid progress on a new exercise throughout your workouts. You start at a low level, far below your potential strength.

For someone who is not accustomed to strength-building movements, it is difficult to reach the critical threshold of intensity necessary for rapid growth. As a beginner, the best way to increase intensity is to know that you did 10 crunches during the previous workout and that you must do at least 11 today with proper form.

If you change exercises too frequently, your muscles will not have the time to learn how to work hard on the old exercise. All the time spent learning a new exercise is actually time lost as far as aesthetic improvements are concerned. Changing exercises frequently when it is not necessary multiplies these nonproductive periods of motor learning.

Disadvantages of a Single Exercise

Some athletes feel the need to do as many abdominal and core exercises as possible during a workout. If this describes you, then go ahead and do it! These people will quickly grow bored if they are doing only a single exercise. Motivation and enthusiasm diminish along with the joy of working out, which eventually leads to an untenable situation. For these reasons, you must account for psychological factors (such as the desire to keep things fresh and new).

Choosing Variety: An Advanced Strategy

If, after three to five sets of the same exercise, your strength is gone and you are bored, you should do one of two things:

1. Choose a second exercise.
2. End the workout.

If your enthusiasm and strength are renewed when you do the second exercise, then this is the best strategy. If your strength decreases even more during the second exercise, then that is a sign that it is better to stay there. At that point, it is clear that you should stick to a single exercise.

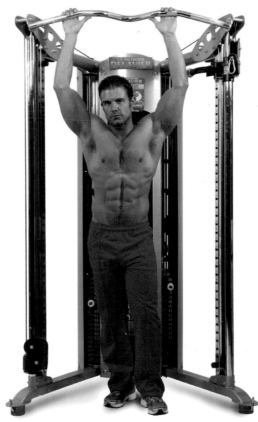

9 When should you change exercises?

As your muscles grow, you must constantly change your program. Beginners will make progress easily, even and especially by following the same exercise program week after week. While the same routine is producing good results, you should really keep doing it. Changing the structure of your program too often creates negative interference. It slows motor learning and prevents you from increasing the intensity of your efforts over time. However, when you notice your progress stalls over several consecutive workouts, then it is time to modify your workout program. The first adjustment you should make is to the types of exercises.

OVERTRAINING: AN ISSUE OF THE NERVOUS SYSTEM

At some point, you might realize that you felt strong and comfortable doing a certain exercise, but now you feel weak when doing it. You cannot really feel the exercise anymore.

The reason for this reversal is that if you perform the same exercise every time you work out, you can end up "frying" your neuromuscular circuit. In fact, every exercise uses a unique connection between the nerves (which control contraction) and the muscle (which performs the movement). By using the same neuromuscular circuit repeatedly, you can eventually wear it out. This local fatigue shows itself through the loss of good sensations when doing that particular exercise. This signals that it is past time for a radical change in your abdominal and core exercises.

10 How many repetitions should you do per set?

> DEFINITION: The number of repetitions is the total number of times you perform a given exercise in a set (see the definition on page 12). There are three stages in a repetition:
> 1. Positive stage: You lift your torso, your legs, or a weight using your abdominal and core muscles.
> 2. Static stage: You maintain the contracted position of the muscles for a few seconds.
> 3. Negative stage: You slowly lower the weight using your abdominal and core muscles.

It is perfectly normal to wonder how many repetitions you should do in a set. But you should know that there is no magic number of repetitions that will determine the quality of your results.

More than repetitions, what really counts is the intensity of the muscle contraction. Changing the number of repetitions is only one method of progressing, not an end in itself. Still, it is good to change the number of repetitions to suit your goals.

Goal: Strengthen Your Core

As a general rule, you can strengthen your core by doing 12 to 15 repetitions. But if you can do 16 repetitions at a given weight instead of 15, then do it! In the next set, however, you should use a heavier weight.

Warning: It is not worthwhile to do fewer than 8 repetitions when working your abdominal and core muscles.

Goal: Lose Inches Off Your Waist

To slim down your waist, you need to do a higher number of repetitions. You should do 20 to 50 repetitions.

Goal: Get a Cardio Workout Using Abdominal and Core Exercises

For endurance and cardiovascular health, you should do circuits of at least 50 repetitions, and you could even do more than 100.

Your workout could very well consist of a combination of these repetition brackets. For example, to get a six-pack and lose inches at the same time, 3 sets of 12 repetitions could be followed by 3 sets of 50 repetitions.

Alternatively, a workout could be based on heavy weights (doing fewer than 15 repetitions) while the subsequent workout could be dedicated to losing inches using long sets (50 to 100 repetitions). In this way, you will have more rest days between two strenuous workouts, which will enhance your recovery.

Goal: Improve Your Athletic Performance

Your chosen number of repetitions should match the duration of effort required by your sport. So in sports requiring explosiveness over a short period (sprinting, throwing, jumping), follow the guidelines for strengthening your core.

For endurance activities, follow the guidelines for cardio work. For activities that fall somewhere in between endurance and explosiveness, follow the guidelines for cardio work.

You could also be more specific by using a blend of strength and endurance work. For example, in group sports (such as soccer and rugby) where both sprinting and endurance are necessary, try alternating strengthening core workouts with cardio core workouts.

PYRAMID GROWTH

You can visualize training your abdominal and core muscles as a pyramid. You must start with light resistance and lots of repetitions (25, for example, that are easy for you to do) to warm up the muscles thoroughly and give you a good cardiorespiratory warm-up too.

For the second set, increase the weight so that you can easily do 15 repetitions. These two warm-up sets precondition your body.

Now it is time to get serious: Add resistance so that you are targeting 12 repetitions. But as we have said, never stop a set just because you have reached your desired number of repetitions (except during a warm-up). The more repetitions you do at a given weight, the more intensely your muscles will contract. This will help you progress more quickly.

Gradually increase the resistance as you do more sets (thereby increasing the difficulty of the exercise). For the last set of your workout, you can either use the heaviest weight possible or you can lower the weight to really get the blood moving in your muscles. Generally people prefer one of these two strategies. You can also end one workout with heavy weights and end the next workout with light weights.

11 How quickly should you perform repetitions?

As just described, a repetition consists of three distinct stages. To learn how to master muscle contractions well, it is best to start by moving the weight or your body relatively slowly.

The worst thing you can do as a beginner is to swing your torso or your legs wildly while twisting and arching your back. This will create bad habits that are difficult to break later on. At best, cheating will slow your progress. At worst, you could injure yourself! When in doubt, slow down the exercise instead of doing it quickly. However, you can adjust the speed of the repetitions to suit your goals.

Goal: Strengthen Your Core

To get a great six-pack, you have to lift the weight using the strength of your muscles, and you cannot move too quickly:

1. Take 2 to 3 seconds to lift the weight, the torso, or the legs.
2. Hold the contracted position for 2 seconds while contracting your abdominal and core muscles as much as possible.
3. Lower in 2 seconds.

A repetition should therefore take 6 to 7 seconds in total. Even if you can do more repetitions by moving faster, you will be using inertia and not the strength in your abdominal and core muscles.

When you reach fatigue during a set, give yourself a break for 1 to 2 seconds in the lengthened position. Relax your muscles as much as possible so they can rest and temporarily regain their strength. This way, you will be able to do a few more repetitions.

Goal: Lose Inches Off Your Waist

In this case, you should perform repetitions slightly faster to increase your energy and maintain continuous tension in your muscles:

1. Take 2 (true) seconds to lift the weight, torso, or legs.
2. Hold the contracted position for 1 second while contracting your abdominal and core muscles.
3. Relax slowly and lower in 1 to 2 seconds.

So a repetition should take 4 to 5 seconds in total. When you lose strength, take a brief rest in the lengthened position so that you will be able to do a few more repetitions.

Goal: Get a Cardio Workout Using Abdominal and Core Exercises

To increase your repetitions, you will need to use your body's inertia a little bit more, but without going overboard. Each repetition will be done rather energetically:

1. Take 1 second to lift the weight, torso, or legs.
2. Do not hold the contracted position. Immediately start lowering the weight once you have reached the height of the movement.
3. Lower in 1 second.

A repetition should therefore take 2 seconds in total. The abdominal and core muscles remain contracted throughout. When the burning becomes unbearable, give yourself a short break by taking a few seconds of rest in the relaxed position. Once the burning is gone, start again until you have regained the intensity. Take a short break again, and then start again, and so on.

Goal: Improve Your Athletic Performance

The speed with which you perform exercises should match the speed required by your sport. For a sport that requires explosiveness, you should work dynamically:

1. Take less than 1 second to lift the weight, torso, or legs.
2. Do not hold the contracted position.
3. Lower in less than 1 second.

For endurance sports, you could do the exercise more slowly, but use continuous tension:

1. Take 1 to 2 seconds to lift the weight, torso, or legs.
2. Do not hold the contracted position.
3. Lower in less than 1 second.

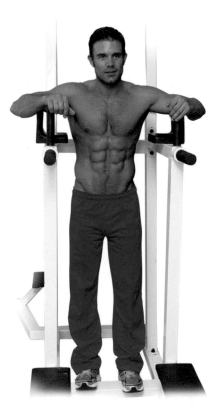

12 Adjust range of motion in the exercises.

The range of motion in the exercises should be adjusted to suit your goals. How far you move can vary greatly during an exercise. If the range of contraction in the abdominal and core muscles is relatively short, it is possible to increase it in the following ways:

- Stretch your torso using a prop or a stability ball that you put under your lumbar spine.
- Enhance the flexibility of the spine by doing exercises on a relatively soft surface (stability ball or mattress) rather than on the floor.
- Work the hip flexors rather than the abdominal and core muscles, which allows you to completely lift the torso or legs. This technique is the most dangerous and the least effective.

Goal: Strengthen Your Core

The range of motion will be greater here. To be able to increase the weight you are using as you do more sets, you need to reduce your range of motion progressively while pulling less on your abdominal and core muscles at the beginning of the exercise. However, do not shorten the range of motion during the contraction stage. If you do, the exercise will be less effective because you will be trying to use too much weight.

Goal: Lose Inches Off Your Waist

The range of motion will be somewhat reduced here, especially at the beginning of the exercise (lengthened position), so that you can maintain continuous tension. As you do more sets, you can slightly restrict the contracted position in order to get a few more repetitions.

Goal: Get a Cardio Workout Using Abdominal and Core Exercises

It is good to maintain as much continuous tension as possible in your abdominal and core muscles, which also means the range of motion here will be the smallest. You should not completely lower your torso or legs. Keep them as high as possible, even if you cannot reach the maximum position.

Goal: Improve Your Athletic Performance

Your range of motion in the exercise should match what is required by your sport. So, if you are a javelin thrower, you should work on increasing the stretch at the beginning of the exercise because you need to have power even while the torso is leaning backward. The same is true if you are a swimmer specializing in the butterfly, because you need strength even while your back is arched.

The opposite is true in cycling, where you need to lift your legs high in the contracted position without having to go very far in the lengthened position.

Runners, and particularly sprinters, must lift the legs high in the contracted position while at the same time trying to increase the stretch at the beginning of the exercise. This means maximum range of motion in the exercises.

In sports requiring rotation (such as golf and the freestyle stroke in swimming), the focus is on the range of motion in the obliques rather than in the abdominal muscles. This is to prevent injuries caused by abruptly stretching obliques that are not very flexible.

How long should a workout last?

The goal of a good workout is to stimulate the muscles to their maximum in the shortest time possible. We are careful to favor a workout's intensity rather than its length.

The very first criteria that determine the duration of your workout are your schedule and your availability. If you do not have a lot of time, you should know that it is possible to do a nonstop core circuit in less than 5 minutes. Still, it is better to take at least 10 minutes for a workout, and we do not recommend working out for more than 20 minutes. If it takes longer than that, then one or more of these conditions is true:

- You are doing too many exercises.
- You are doing too many sets.
- You are taking too much rest time between sets.

The length of your workout will depend on two things:

- The amount of work (number of exercises plus number of sets)
- The amount of rest between sets

You will have to play around with the rest time between sets if you do not have enough time for your workouts.

WHY DO YOU NEED TO WARM UP?

Your body is like a car. If you accelerate quickly when the motor is cold, you will not go much faster, and you could damage the mechanical parts in the engine. But when the motor is warm, just a slight acceleration will quickly increase your speed. Just like a car, your muscles can work their hardest only at a certain temperature. This is why it is essential that you warm up before any exercise. Warming up will give you the following benefits:

1. Protect you from injury
2. Optimize your performance
3. Help you mentally prepare for the work ahead

⚠ The length of your warm-up can vary depending on the season and the time of day. For example, in the winter or in the early morning, your body is colder than in the summer or in the afternoon. This means you will need to add one or two sets to your warm-up. The rest of your workout does not necessarily need to be shortened, so your total workout time will automatically be a little bit longer.

14 How much rest time should you take between sets?

The rest time between sets can vary from 1 second to 1 minute, depending on the difficulty of the exercise as well as your goals. You should take

- more rest after difficult exercises like hanging leg raises or sit-ups,
- less rest after easier exercises like crunches,
- more rest when you are using heavier resistance, and
- less rest when you are using light resistance.

As a general rule, it is time to add another set when

- your breathing is almost back to normal, and
- you feel like your enthusiasm is overcoming any fatigue.

However, before beginning a new set, be sure that you are focused again:

- Know how many repetitions you have done.
- Focus once more on your goals.

At first, time yourself so that you adhere to the rest time you decided on. Timing yourself will help you be rigorous and avoid taking rest breaks that are too long. Keeping track of the time will also help you control the intensity and duration of your workout. Your goal should be to adjust your rest time more precisely.

⚠ If you start to lose strength abnormally from one set to the next, it is for one of these reasons:

- You have done too many sets.
- You have not rested long enough.

In this second case, you can try slightly increasing your rest time to see if that resolves the problem. If that does not work, it means the duration of the rest was not responsible for the decrease in performance. You simply did too many sets.

Goal: Strengthen Your Core

If you want to strengthen your muscles, it is not a good idea to restrict your rest time too much. You need to allow your muscles the time they require to recover their strength completely. Heavily working a muscle that is not fully recovered is counterproductive. But you should not totally relax and fall asleep during your workout, either. A good average for a rest break is 45 seconds to 1 minute. But a rest break lasting more than 2 minutes between sets is too long.

Goal: Lose Inches Off Your Waist

Rest breaks between sets should be relatively brief: no longer than 30 seconds. A good strategy is to reduce your rest time progressively with each workout while striving to maintain (or even increase) your repetitions. For example, if you have done a workout with 30 seconds of rest time between sets, try to repeat that effort while taking only 25 seconds of rest. If, after several sets, you cannot keep up that pace, then increase your rest time to 30 seconds. During the next workout, try to do even more sets (or possibly the whole workout) with only 25 seconds of rest between sets.

Goal: Get a Cardio Workout Using Abdominal and Core Exercises

The ideal method here is to do circuits. That is, do different exercises one after the other with no real rest time in between. The only respite is during the transition from one exercise to the next. Throughout the workout, as the circuits become more and more difficult to accomplish, you can give yourself a 10-second break between each exercise.

Goal: Improve Your Athletic Performance

You should calculate your rest time based on the requirements for your sport. Thus, in sports with brief but intense explosive movements, follow the guidelines previously given for strengthening your core. In sports requiring both endurance and explosiveness, such as team sports, follow the guidelines previously given for losing inches off your waist. For pure endurance sports, follow the cardio model.

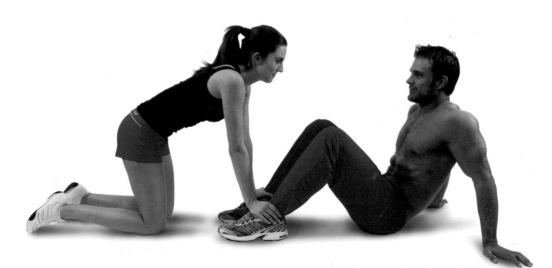

15 Determine the most appropriate weight for each exercise.

More than the number of repetitions or sets, the resistance (or weight) that you use in each exercise determines the effectiveness of your training. You must use a weight that is appropriate for your strength.

In the beginning, it might be difficult to figure out which weight to use. With no weight, certain exercises are too easy while others might seem impossible to do. You will go back and forth a bit, but this is not wasted time. It helps you develop something called muscle memory. All the difficulties in this selection process are because it is not natural to have to select a resistance to impose on your muscles.

In nature, muscle work adapts to the weight, not the other way around. For example, when you run, your stride automatically adapts to the difficulty of the terrain. In strength training, the logic is reversed. It is as if you were adapting the terrain to the type of stride you wish to have. Your brain and central nervous system have to get used to this paradoxical logic. The process is further complicated when you add in your ever-present desire to use weights that are too heavy in the hopes of reaching your goals faster.

To find the right resistance for each exercise, start with a light weight and gradually increase it. There are three broad weight zones:

- Zone 1 involves light weights that do not require much effort to lift.
- Zone 2 involves weights that allow you to both perform the exercise correctly and feel your muscles working.
- Zone 3 involves weights that require you to cheat in order to lift and do not let you feel your muscles working.

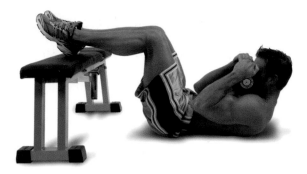

The process for selecting resistance begins with the warm-up. A good warm-up will help you calibrate the level of resistance for your abdominal and core muscles. You must always start with a light weight. First, do a warm-up set with a weight in the middle of zone 1. For the second warm-up set, use a weight from the upper part of zone 1.

Three-quarters of your working sets should be done with weights from zone 2, gradually increasing the weight with each set (the pyramid strategy; see page 15). This increase should take you from the lower part of zone 2 to the upper part.

You can do one last set with weights from the lower part of zone 3. Handling a weight that is a little too heavy prepares the central nervous system for the next workout. This technique, called intrusion, increases intensity. But you should never abuse this strategy!

> ⚠ Telling you that the weight should be different for each exercise does not really help. Once you have found the correct weight for an exercise, write it down in your notebook (see page 24) along with the number of repetitions you did. During your next workout, try to do one or two more repetitions at the same weight.

16 When should you increase the weight?

The weight that you can use for each exercise is constantly changing. In the best case, your strength increases and you can use heavier and heavier weights. But the natural tendency is to want to skip ahead of this gain in strength and increase the weight too quickly. This means your form deteriorates progressively during exercises and you feel less work happening in your abs. You can end up losing your motivation because your

workouts become more and more arduous. Knowing how and when to increase the weight is a critical factor for progress. To decide if your muscles are ready for more resistance, you can use two criteria:

- **Number of repetitions:** When you reach your target number of repetitions (15 for strengthening muscles or 50 for losing inches off your waist, for example), it is time to ask yourself if you need to increase your weight.

- **Ease in handling the weight:** In reaching the target number, did your form deteriorate? There are generally two scenarios. To increase the weight at the right moment, you must absolutely be in the second scenario:

1. You have artificially reached your target number. There is a natural tendency to cheat more and more to convince yourself that you are making progress. In this case, wait one or two workouts, during which you try to do the exercise with perfect form rather than change the weight.

2. You feel very comfortable with a weight that seems too light. In this case, definitely increase the weight. Increase the weight proportionally to the number of additional repetitions you did beyond your target number. If you exceeded your goal by one or two repetitions, then you only need to add a small amount of weight. In general, the smallest amount you can increase your weight is one or two pounds. It is not a good idea to increase at a faster rate unless you have really blown by your target number. In this case only, you can make a bigger increase.

Don't Go Too Fast!

There is an additional difficulty when working the abdominal and core muscles. The more you increase the resistance (by adding weight or putting weight plates on a machine), the farther the center of gravity for the exercise will shift. This shifting will progressively reduce the participation of the abs and recruit the hip flexors instead. This is why you can really feel a light exercise in your abs, but when you add a little bit of weight, you can no longer feel the abs working.

Similarly, sometimes just a little bit more weight can really affect your technique in performing the exercise. It is better to increase the weight slightly and more often than to do it abruptly and then require several workouts to rediscover the sensations.

If you decide to ignore these warnings and skip ahead, you will be moving the weight less and less with your abs. You will be using more inertia from momentum or twisting. This puts you at risk for injury, which will delay your progress even more.

Change Your Warm-Up!

The stronger you get and the heavier the weight you can use during the first set, the more critical your warm-up becomes. When you are not very strong, the joints, muscles, and tendons do not need a lot of warming up since a lot of tension is not required. But as you progress, it is good to increase the amount of warm-up sets because the tension you put on your muscles is getting closer to their breaking point.

17 Determine rest time between exercises.

It is not necessary to increase your rest time between two exercises. With the exception of circuits, catch your breath by taking the same amount of rest that you took between sets. If you feel tired, take a longer break, especially at the end of a workout. You still need to keep doing the exercises close together to keep your muscles warm, remain focused, and avoid having a never-ending workout.

When you are circuit training, you should not take breaks between exercises. Ideally, between two circuits, you should limit yourself to a brief rest break or even skip it altogether.

When you get tired after a few circuits, you can start taking 15 to 30 seconds of rest so that you can complete one or two more circuits.

18 Learn to choose exercises that work for you.

In this book, we have carefully selected the most effective abdominal and core exercises. However, not all of the exercises will necessarily suit you. This is because individual body types vary tremendously. You might be very tall, or very short, or average height. Your legs might be very long or very short in relation to your torso. Or your torso might be very long or very short.

Each body type requires individualized exercise choices. We would be lying if we said that all body types could adapt to any exercise. Certain builds are just better suited for some exercises.

There are two complementary ways to select your exercises:

- **By elimination:** Some exercises do not work well with your anatomy. You should eliminate those first off. Other exercises do not match your goals. These two parameters restrict the possibilities and, therefore, make your choices easier. However, simple elimination should not be your only criterion in making a decision. It is better to find exercises that work for you.
- **By selection:** To determine compatibility between your body type and an exercise, often the only way is to try the exercise. You will find some exercises that you like right away. But most of the time you will find them a bit strange, and you will have difficulty doing them since they involve muscles that you are not accustomed to using. With time, the novelty will fade and you will feel the contraction in your abdominal and core muscles more and more.

Learn to Differentiate Between Exercises

Your choice will be easier once you understand that there are differences between exercises. You should learn to recognize the differences and use them to your advantage. So each exercise has both advantages and disadvantages. Only by mastering the concept of advantages and disadvantages will you find exercises whose advantages best meet your needs and disadvantages contradict your goals the least.

For this reason, we are particularly attentive in describing the advantages and disadvantages of each exercise in parts 3, 4, and 5 of this book. From there, you will have a solid and logical base to choose from.

A Situation in Constant Evolution

As far as the choice of exercises goes, it is important not to get stuck in a rut. With time, you will learn to appreciate certain exercises that you did not like before. When this happens, you might regret that you did not realize this sooner. You might feel as if you have lost some time. But this is rarely true. Muscle sensations are constantly changing. A month or two ago, perhaps your abdominal and core muscles were not ready for that exercise. The progress you have made means that you can now feel that new exercise. So you should not have any regrets.

The opposite can also happen: You feel less and less from an exercise that you especially liked before. This exercise guaranteed rapid progress at first, but it has now become ineffective. This is not just a feeling. It means that it is past time to remove this exercise from your program. After several weeks of not doing this exercise, you can try to reintroduce it.

You must continually adapt to your changing muscles and not be too rigid in dealing with those changes. This commonsense observation might make you wonder how to determine when it is time to change your workout program.

19 Know when to change your workout program.

Some people need to do the same thing and keep repeating the same workout program. This is easy to understand. After all, once you have found something that works, why change it? Other people require novelty. It is impossible to know beforehand which group you belong to, and the majority of people are probably somewhere in the middle. But, in general, your state of mind rather accurately reflects your muscles' needs. There are two objective criteria that signal it is time to change your workout routine:

- **Plateau or loss of strength:** When your progress abruptly stops, it means that something is no longer working. We are not talking about one or two poor workouts, but a trend over at least one week. A radical change is required at this time.
- **Boredom:** When you lose enthusiasm for working your core, it means that your program is too monotonous. It is time for something new! There are two kinds of boredom, and you have to figure out which is affecting you because they do not require the same number of changes to your program. We begin with the kind of boredom that requires the most changes to your program and end with the kind that requires only subtle changes in your training program.

1. Great boredom or even a complete lack of interest in working the core. This generally means you have been overtraining. In this case, it is time to take a break or reduce the amount of work you do. The best solution here is to completely restructure your workout program.
2. Lack of interest in an exercise. This is a sign that you have burned out the specific neuromuscular pathway for that exercise. You have to replace that exercise, but you may not need to make any other changes.

Conclusion

There is no set rule for how often you should modify your workout program. As long as your workouts are giving you regular results, why change them? There will always come a time when you will feel the need to make changes. Your muscles will let you know by drastically reducing their rate of progress. The difference between a beginner and an experienced athlete is how quickly you perceive these signals. So be attentive and be sure to keep a notebook (see page 24) so that you can quickly pick up on these clues.

20 Taking a vacation?

You could certainly train year-round, but that is not necessarily a good strategy for long-term progress. It is a good idea to take a few weeks off every year. This way, while you are resting your body, your mind, muscles, and joints have a chance to recover. Just as you have to take a step back before you can jump as far as possible, taking a break could help you make it past a point that once seemed impossible to reach.

All the same, there are three inconveniences involved in taking a vacation:

- Strength and endurance will diminish, but you will quickly regain your previous level. However, the longer the break you take, the harder it will be to gain back your previous level.
- Frequently, a week's vacation becomes several weeks, months, and then years. Taking a break and then starting again require discipline that many people do not have. For some people, it is better never to stop exercising, because they might never start again.

UNDERSTANDING MUSCULAR DECONDITIONING

The central nervous system is the first part of your body that responds to exercise, and it is also the first affected by deconditioning during rest periods. Loss of strength can therefore be rapid. Fortunately, muscle is more resistant to weakening, so a decrease in strength after a couple weeks of vacation does not mean you have lost muscle. Do not worry, because your central nervous system will regain its efficiency within a few workouts.

- Often, interrupting your exercise means increasing calorie intake, while the reverse is preferable. When you are not exercising, you must be aware of your food intake or you will end up gaining weight.

Keep a Workout Notebook

It is very important to keep a workout notebook. It immediately helps you see what you did during your previous core workout. Make a small box where you can note the time you start your workout. Below that, write down when you finished. This way you will know exactly how much time you spent exercising. Measuring the time spent is an important factor, because if you rest longer between sets, your performance will increase but you won't necessarily get stronger. To truly compare two workouts, you must ensure they are approximately the same length.

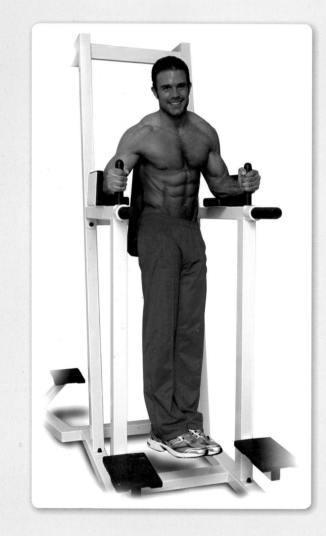

Your workout notebook should be as precise as possible but still easy to maintain. Here is an example:

> Crunch with a dumbbell on the chest:
> — 5 lbs: 20 reps
> — 10 lbs: 17 reps
> — 15 lbs: 13 reps
> — 20 lbs: 8 reps
> Time: 5 min.

We know which exercise was done (crunch), the weight, the number of repetitions, the number of sets, and how much time it took.

Do the same for all workouts. This is how you will determine exactly what your goals are for your next workout.

Analyze Your Workouts

After each workout, analyze your performance by asking yourself these questions:

- What worked well?
- What did not work well?
- Why did it not work well?
- How can I make things better during my next workout?

If you look at the previous example, here is a typical analysis you could do for each exercise before your next workout:

- Start with a heavier weight because the first set might be too light (you did 20 repetitions).
- Carry this same increase in weight over to the second as well as the third sets.
- In the third set, the muscles start to get tired, because you lost four repetitions instead of three for an increase of 5 pounds in weight. You will have to stick with it to overcome this fatigue.

- In the last set, the loss of strength is accentuated with a loss of five repetitions for an additional 5 pounds. You must halt the rate at which you are increasing the weight so that you will be able to do more repetitions using a lower weight than last time. The new workout would look like this:

Crunch with a dumbbell on the chest:
- — 10 lbs: 18 reps
- — 15 lbs: 15 reps
- — 17.5 lbs: 12 reps
- — 20 lbs: 10 reps
Time: 5 min.

For the next workout, your goal will be to increase the number of repetitions using the same amount of weight. Increase the weight again once you reach 20 repetitions.

How Do You Finish Your Analysis?

The trend over a month, rather than from one workout to another, is what helps you adjust your core workout program. If your numbers are increasing regularly, then all is well! If your increase slows down, you can change things by doing the following:

- Switching exercises
- Resting more between workouts

If you notice a persistent loss of strength, then you need to both lower the weight and increase your rest time.

Conclusion

Only a well-maintained workout notebook can precisely show how your performance has changed over time. Do not just rely on your memory. Of course you can remember the numbers from your last workout. But how will you remember what you did a month ago? Also, if you change exercises, how will you remember what you did for that exercise when you introduce it again one or two months later? Your workout notebook is the best way to monitor your progress, and it is an important aid in creating future workout programs.

Making Progress

The very first effects of a core workout are stiff muscles. This trauma inflicted on your muscle fibers is a wake-up call that will be more or less painful depending on your physical fitness level. To hasten your recovery, it is okay to work out again lightly.

After your stiff muscles have recovered, your strength and endurance will quickly progress. In fact, the central nervous system adapts to this new environment. It will learn to coordinate muscle efforts better by allowing different groups of fibers to work in harmony with each other.

Strength might develop more quickly than your muscles, but they will eventually become more toned. But as we see every day, it is difficult to judge your daily progress. This is why you might feel stuck. And then, one day, you realize that you need to tighten your belt a notch.

As long as you are working out on a regular basis, your muscles will ultimately react. However, it is impossible to know how fast they will react because everyone develops at a different rate.

So that you can more easily see your transformation, take a photo of yourself at least once a month and measure the circumference of your waist every week. Your muscles will be noticeable even faster if you stick to a lower-calorie diet in addition to working out regularly.

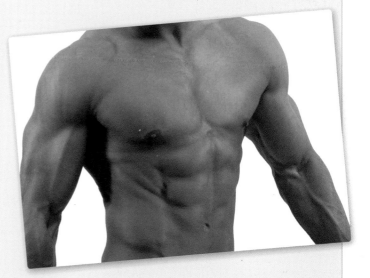

PART 2

Increase the Visibility of Your Abs

There is no point in having good abdominal muscles if they are covered by a thick layer of fat. In addition to strengthening your ab muscles, it is a good idea to enhance their visibility. The three weapons at your disposal are exercise, diet, and nutritional supplements.

Exercising Your Abs for a Smaller Waist

A common belief is that there is no point in working your abs if you are not on a calorie-restricted diet.

This is largely true for a sedentary person who is overweight. If you have more than 15 percent body fat, you won't see a six-pack. Working your ab muscles will not change anything!

But when the body fat percentage is reasonable (around 10 percent), regularly working your abdominal muscles will make a huge difference for these reasons:

1. If you never work your abdominal muscles, they never have a chance to become toned. Abdominal muscles that are not really toned are relatively smooth. A thin layer of fat is enough to hide them.
2. On the contrary, the more toned your abdominal muscles are, the more visible they will be, even with a high percentage of fat.
3. Scientific research by Stallknecht et al. in 2007 (*American Journal of Physiology—Endocrinology and Metabolism* 292(2): E394-9) shows that a contracting muscle gets part of its energy from the fat covering it.
4. Even without a calorie-restricted diet or weight loss, it is possible to trim fat from the waist by doing regular physical activity (Lee et al., 2005. *Journal of Applied Physiology* 99:1220-5). In fact, exercise helps localize fat loss around the waist (see the following section titled Intensity First!).
5. Your body stores fat first on your least active muscles. By regularly working your abs, you reduce the chance that fat will accumulate on your belly.

Conclusion

Regularly working your abdominal muscles has two benefits. It helps fight fat locally and tones the rectus abdominis, which enhances its visibility.

Intensity First!

Medical research by Irving et al. in 2008 (*Medicine and Science in Sports and Exercise* 40(11): 1863-72) shows that, when the same number of calories is burned, the intensity of the exercise has a strong effect on localizing fat loss in the abdominal area. For example, over a period of 16 weeks, overweight women exercised five times per week without following a low-calorie diet. Part of the group did their exercise with high intensity while the others trained with low intensity.

Even though the two types of exercise burned the same number of calories (400), fat loss was twice as great when the exercise was done at high intensity (6 pounds [2.8 kg]) than when it was done at low intensity (3 pounds [1.3 kg]). Only high-intensity training resulted in an 8.5 percent loss of belly fat. No reduction was noted for low-intensity exercise. High-intensity exercise is superior because of its deferred metabolic effects: Long after you stop exercising, your body will still burn calories. Strength training with the highest intensity possible is the perfect way to get rid of your love handles.

Diet as a Way to Slim Your Waist

Nutrition plays primarily an accelerating role in eliminating belly fat. But restricting calories alone is not always effective in revealing your abdominal muscles. On the contrary, some people on a diet feel as though they are gaining belly fat.

A medical study led by You et al. in 2005 (*American Journal of Physiology—Endocrinology and Metabolism* 288: E741-7) illustrates this phenomenon perfectly. In five months on a low-calorie diet, women saw the size of their abdominal fat cells increase by 5 percent.

This paradox is easily explained. When the body experiences calorie deprivation, it mobilizes a large amount of lipids from fatty tissue. It burns only one-third of this fat at most. This means the other two-thirds are redeposited in fatty areas. Furthermore, lipids are stored first in the "calmest" areas—that is, places not disturbed by intense blood circulation.

This physiological characteristic explains why your body stores fat first on muscles that are not frequently used, such as the abdominal muscles or the buttocks. Unless a person is truly obese, it is rare to have a lot of fat on the forearms or the calves (these muscles are frequently used, which activates blood flow in those areas).

Diet Plus Workout Synergy

The You et al. study (2005) describes a synergy between consuming a low-calorie diet and exercising the abs. Dieting alone increased belly fat, but when that same diet was coupled with regular physical activity, the size of the fat cells on the abs decreased by 10 percent.

Types of Abdominal Walls

① Normal abdominal wall, with toned muscles.
② Normal abdominal wall, with toned muscles and a layer of subcutaneous fat that gives the impression of a ptosis.*
③ Abdominal wall with a ptosis due to lack of muscle tone, with no layer of fat.
④ Abdominal wall with a ptosis due to lack of muscle tone, accompanied by a layer of fat.

*Ptosis is a downward movement of an organ most often caused by a weakening of the structures that maintain it. When the abdominal wall lacks tone, it can no longer hold back the viscera. The belly sinks and forms a pocket where the intestinal loops end up.

SUBCUTANEOUS FAT AND VISCERAL FAT

The abdominal muscles, without necessarily being dry, are not usually covered by as much fat as you might think. Unless you are truly obese, the view of your rectus abdominis is only obscured by perhaps an inch of fat. The thickness of this fat only rarely reaches five inches. Often, a potbelly is not caused by this subcutaneous fat. Instead, it comes from the inside, from what is called visceral fat. This is internal fat that pushes the abdomen outward.

Improving the Effectiveness of Your Diet

Low-carbohydrate diets are the most effective at accentuating the loss of inches off the waist. In fact, eating sugar, as well as alcohol, promotes belly fat. It is a good idea to moderate your consumption of bread, pasta, rice, candy, and pastries.

Pay special attention to sweetened soda, because it is rich in both sugar and caffeine. In fact, caffeine promotes the absorption of sugar, making it even more harmful to your health and your figure.

On the contrary, decaffeinated coffee is rich in chlorogenic acid, which reduces the absorption of carbohydrate, and can be advantageously used at the end of a meal.

Role of Supplements

Supplements such as BCAA and calcium help to localize the loss of fat off the waist.

BCAAs for Losing Belly Fat

What Are BCAAs?

BCAAs (branched-chain amino acids) are made up of three essential amino acids: leucine, isoleucine, and valine. By themselves, these amino acids make up one-third of all muscle proteins. However, your body does not have the enzymes required for synthesizing the acids. You can provide the BCAAs your body needs only through diet or supplementation.

How Do BCAAs Work?
BCAAs

- promote muscle strengthening;
- fight the accumulation of fat;
- stimulate the natural secretion of growth hormone, an anti-fat hormone that tones muscles;
- support the secretion of leptin, a hormone that stops hunger;
- fight physical and mental fatigue during exercise and while dieting.

Results

For three weeks, athletes followed a specific diet (1,800 calories per day) more or less rich in protein and BCAAs:

- A diet that was low in protein (15 percent of calorie intake) and low in BCAAs resulted in a total loss of 4.2 pounds [1.9 kg].
- A high-protein diet (25 percent of intake) that was low in BCAAs (9 g per day) resulted in a loss of 5.3 pounds [2.4 kg].
- A diet with an average amount of protein (20 percent of intake) but rich in BCAAs (35 g per day) resulted in a loss of 8.8 pounds [4 kg].

As far as belly fat is concerned

- the low-protein, low-BCAA diet resulted in a loss of 18 percent;
- the high-protein, low-BCAA diet resulted in a loss of 21 percent;
- the moderate-protein diet that was rich in BCAAs resulted in a loss of 27.5 percent.

Conclusion

A diet rich in protein and especially in BCAAs helps to localize fat loss on the abdomen.

How Can You Use BCAAs?

Unless you are eating more protein, a low-calorie diet tends to reduce the level of BCAAs at the very time when you need to increase them. For example, overweight women who followed a diet of 1,000 calories per day for three weeks lost 11 percent of the BCAAs in their bodies.

Branched-chain amino acids can be used in the following forms:

- BCAAs in powder, capsules, or tablets
- Proteins that are highly concentrated in BCAAs (such as whey or casein)

BCAAs can be taken at these times:

- Between meals
- During meals
- Before, during, or just after a workout

While you are on a calorie-restricted diet, it is generally recommended that you take 5 to 10 grams of BCAAs spread out throughout the day. No side effects have been reported, as long as reasonable dosing directions are followed.

Conclusion

While you are on a calorie-restricted diet, BCAAs protect the integrity of your muscles, fight fatigue, and promote fat loss, particularly around the waist.

Calcium: The Anti-Belly Fat Mineral

What Is Calcium?

Calcium is a mineral found in dairy products. It plays a vital role in the health of the bones.

More than a decade ago, no one had made the connection between calcium and weight loss. Only recent scientific discoveries have shown that calcium can help burn fat.

How Does Calcium Work?

When the body lacks calcium, it stores up every little bit it can. One of the places it is stored is inside fat cells. A diet that is poor in calcium causes an increase of this mineral in the fatty tissues, which, in turn, promotes weight gain.

On the contrary, a diet rich in calcium will reduce the concentration of calcium in fat cells. And it is easier to burn fat cells when their growth is inhibited. Calcium's effects on fat are much more noticeable on belly fat.

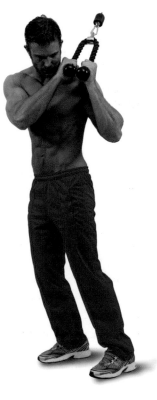

Influence of Calcium Alone

In the 1990s, during studies on high blood pressure, doctors noticed for the first time that increasing calcium from 400 milligrams to 1,000 milligrams per day caused weight loss of about 11 pounds (5 kg) over a year.

Studies show that a person taking less than 500 milligrams of calcium per day is twice as likely to be overweight than someone taking 1,000 milligrams. It is estimated that each 100-milligram increase of calcium translates into a loss of 1.1 pounds [.5 kg] of fat per year. Unfortunately, this beneficial effect does not continue beyond a daily intake of 800 milligrams.

Women benefit more than men from an increase in calcium, undoubtedly because they generally consume less food.

Taking Calcium Supplements While on a Diet

For men and women who eat when they are hungry, calcium intake does not influence the rate of fat breakdown. When these same people lower their intake by 600 calories a day, fat loss is 28 percent greater with an intake of 1.4 grams of calcium than with 500 milligrams (Melanson et al., 2005. *Obesity Research* 13: 2102-12).

Over a period of 6 months, overweight women (average age 38 years) followed a diet of 1,200 to 1,500 calories per day. One group received 1.8 grams of calcium and the other received 1 gram (both groups consumed calcium citrate supplements).

Total fat loss was as follows:

- 6.6 pounds (3 kg) in the 1-gram group
- 11 pounds (5 kg) in the 1.8-gram group

The loss of muscle was 4.4 pounds (2 kg) in the 1-gram group, but it was half that in the other group.

How Should You Use Calcium?

Daily calcium needs vary depending on your age:

- 1.3 grams minimum for adolescents
- 1 gram for adults
- 1.3 grams for people over 50

It is more effective to supplement with calcium in the evening than in the morning. The ideal plan would be to consume two-thirds of your total calcium in the evening and one-third in the morning.

Supplements or Dairy Products?

For weight loss, calcium from dairy products is better than calcium supplements. Unfortunately, including dairy products (milk, yogurt, cheese) in your diet adds calories in the form of fat or sugar.

Different research shows that when these additional calories are consumed in the form of dairy, there is usually no corresponding decrease in intake of other food sources. This noncompensation phenomenon is twice as pronounced in men than in women. It might cancel out the beneficial effects you get from the dairy products to help you lose weight, and this is why supplements tend to be better.

Your total daily calcium intake should not exceed 2.5 grams. Excessive calcium supplementation will not increase weight loss, since the benefits of calcium end well below the 2.5-gram level.

The benefits of calcium and your calcium needs both increase while you are on a calorie-restricted diet. Be sure that your intake meets your needs.

⚠️ **Calcium Intake Is Reduced When You Restrict Calories**

1. The less you eat, the less chance you have of meeting your calcium needs. For example, in women, 6 months on a diet reduces calcium intake by 40% on average.

2. Normally, you assimilate only 25% of your dietary calcium; caloric restrictions lower the rate of assimilation by 15%.

3. Similarly, medical studies show that your calcium needs increase while on a restricted diet.

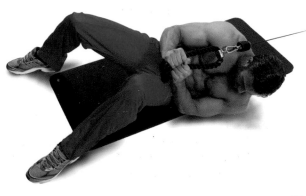

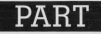

PART 3

Basic Exercises to Sculpt Your Abs

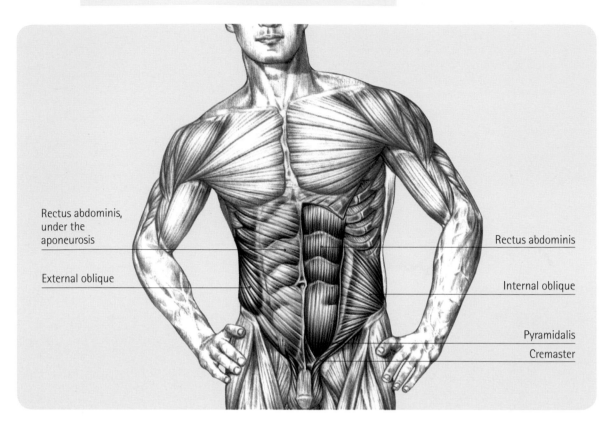

Rectus abdominis, under the aponeurosis

External oblique

Rectus abdominis

Internal oblique

Pyramidalis

Cremaster

Anatomical Considerations

The abdominal wall is made up of four muscles:

1. The rectus abdominis, commonly called the abdominal muscles
2. The external oblique, located on both sides of the rectus abdominis
3. The internal oblique, located under the external oblique
4. The transversus abdominis, located under the obliques

Most people want to get bigger muscles, but muscles on the waist are different. People want definition, not bulk, in that part of the body.

THE MUSCLES IN A SLIM WAIST

The abdominal muscles help hold in the belly, but it is the less well-known muscles that actually make the waist as small as possible:

- The transversus muscle functions as a corset on the waist.
- The external and internal obliques, to a lesser degree, also help refine the abdomen when they are toned but not too muscular.

Action of the abdominal muscles and the system containing the viscera

1. Rectus abdominis
2. External oblique
3. Internal oblique
4. Transversus abdominis

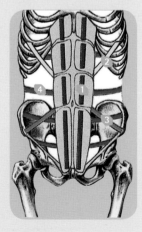

In quadrupeds, the muscles of the abdominal wall passively support the viscera like a hammock. They generally play a relatively limited active role in locomotion. Because humans walk on two feet, the muscles in the abdominal wall are considerably stronger than the abdominal muscles of quadrupeds. In the vertical position, the abdominal muscles stabilize the pelvis with the torso, preventing the latter from swinging too much while walking or running. They have become powerful support muscles, actively sheathing the viscera.

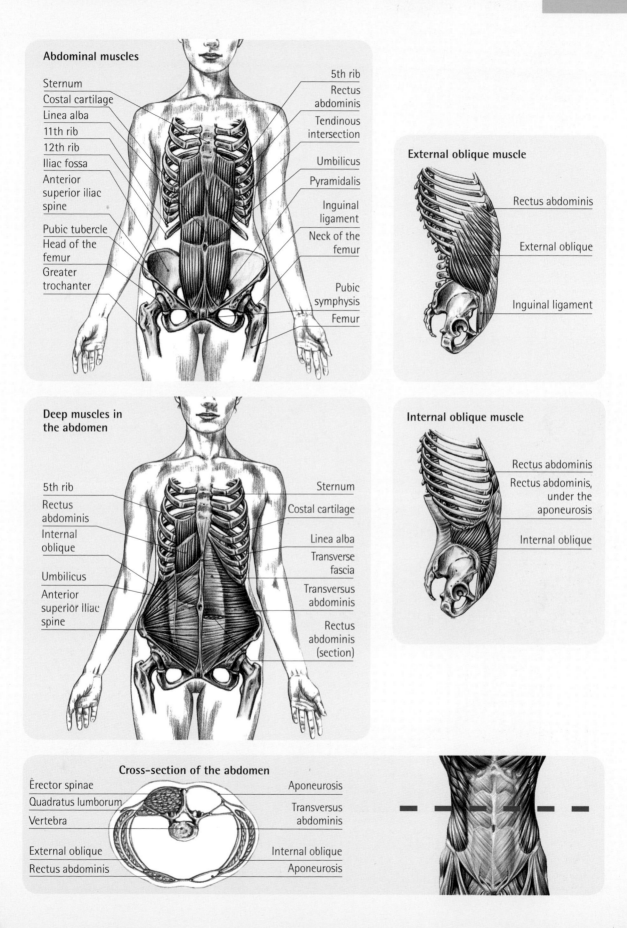

Abdominal muscles

Sternum
Costal cartilage
Linea alba
11th rib
12th rib
Iliac fossa
Anterior superior iliac spine
Pubic tubercle
Head of the femur
Greater trochanter

5th rib
Rectus abdominis
Tendinous intersection
Umbilicus
Pyramidalis
Inguinal ligament
Neck of the femur
Pubic symphysis
Femur

External oblique muscle

Rectus abdominis
External oblique
Inguinal ligament

Deep muscles in the abdomen

5th rib
Rectus abdominis
Internal oblique
Umbilicus
Anterior superior iliac spine

Sternum
Costal cartilage
Linea alba
Transverse fascia
Transversus abdominis
Rectus abdominis (section)

Internal oblique muscle

Rectus abdominis
Rectus abdominis, under the aponeurosis
Internal oblique

Cross-section of the abdomen

Erector spinae
Quadratus lumborum
Vertebra
External oblique
Rectus abdominis

Aponeurosis
Transversus abdominis
Internal oblique
Aponeurosis

35

Beware of Fake Abdominal Exercises!

Unfortunately, there are a lot of fake abdominal exercises out there. They are both ineffective and tiring, and they endanger the spine. But there is an easy way to tell the good exercises from the bad. When the rectus abdominis muscle contracts, it bends the low back. Therefore, any exercise that arches the lumbar spine is not working the abdominal muscles effectively.

The muscles that control the curve of the lower spine are the psoas, iliacus, and rectus femoris. As soon as your lumbar spine comes off the floor, you know that these other muscles are working instead of the abs.

> ⚠ Abdominal exercises exert pressure on the intervertebral discs so that the torso can move forward. This pressure is no problem for a healthy spine, as long as you do the exercise with correct form. If you have back problems or you feel back pain during a workout, you must absolutely consult your doctor so that he or she can determine if you can do these exercises without injuring your back.
>
> Proper abdominal and core exercises aid in the general support of the spine, but fake exercises have the opposite effect. These exercises are useless and dangerous, even for a healthy back.

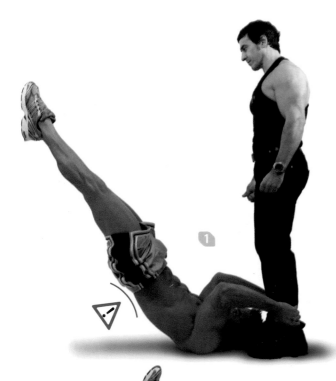

For example, exercises that involve holding your legs in the air for as long as possible ❶ and all scissor-like movements ❷ are kidney breakers. Since the rectus abdominis is attached to the pelvis and not to the thighs, it cannot wiggle the legs. So why are these exercises so painful? Because arching the back is dangerous for the discs, the abdominal muscles try to intervene and straighten the spine. They contract isometrically (that is, without moving), which deprives them of oxygen since their blood circulation is blocked. Large amounts of lactic acid accumulate in the abs since the blood cannot carry it away. This artificial oxygen deprivation causes a local burning sensation. It is a little like running with a plastic bag on your head: You cannot do it for very long. In addition to being dangerous, running without air is counterproductive to good performance. Isometric contraction does not tone the abdominal muscles or help you to lose extra weight.

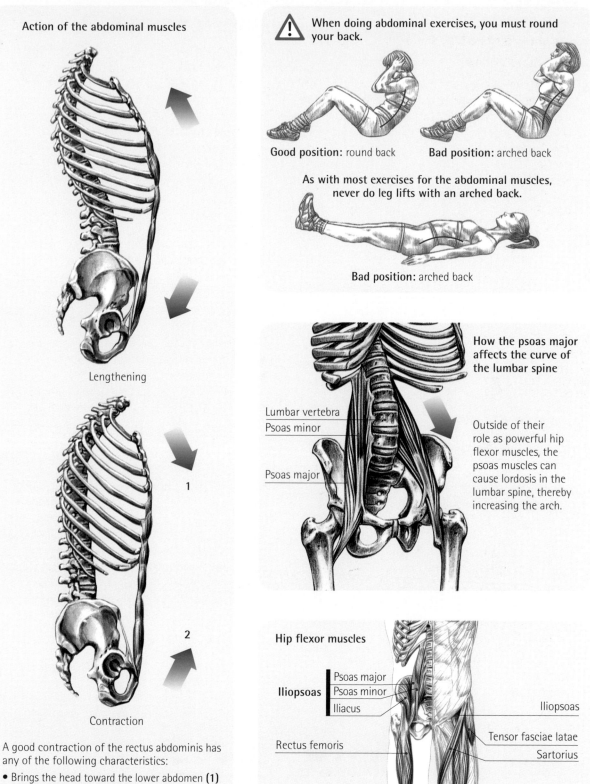

Action of the abdominal muscles

Lengthening

1

2

Contraction

A good contraction of the rectus abdominis has any of the following characteristics:

- Brings the head toward the lower abdomen **(1)**
- Brings the pelvis toward the head **(2)**
- Brings the head and the pelvis simultaneously toward each other **(1 + 2)**

The best exercise here is the crunch.

⚠ When doing abdominal exercises, you must round your back.

Good position: round back   **Bad position:** arched back

As with most exercises for the abdominal muscles, never do leg lifts with an arched back.

Bad position: arched back

How the psoas major affects the curve of the lumbar spine

Lumbar vertebra
Psoas minor

Psoas major

Outside of their role as powerful hip flexor muscles, the psoas muscles can cause lordosis in the lumbar spine, thereby increasing the arch.

Hip flexor muscles

Iliopsoas — Psoas major / Psoas minor / Iliacus

Iliopsoas

Tensor fasciae latae

Sartorius

Rectus femoris

If You Have an Inguinal, Femoral, or Abdominal Hernia

Contrary to popular belief, working your abs will not reduce hernias. Just like torn paper, a hernia cannot repair itself. Exercise could even aggravate the condition. Only a surgeon can repair the hole.

Abdominal and core exercises will not give you a hernia, but if you already have one, they could make it worse. In this case, you should be evaluated by a physician to determine any risks. It is a good idea to seek medical advice not only before you start a core workout program but also before you start any intense physical activity.

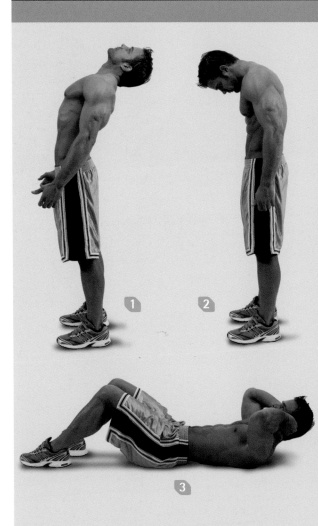

PAY ATTENTION TO THE POSITION OF YOUR HEAD!

The position of your head affects your balance by controlling the contraction of muscles used for posture. When you lean your head back

- the lumbar muscles reflexively contract a bit **1**, and
- the abdominal muscles have a tendency to relax.

When you tilt your head forward,

- the abdominal muscles contract **2**, and
- the lumbar muscles relax.

During an abdominal exercise, the most common error is to look at the ceiling **3**. With your head up, the resulting reflex contraction in the lumbar muscles makes the spine more rigid, thereby preventing a good abdominal contraction.

You also need to avoid moving your head from right to left or left to right. These untimely movements interfere with proper muscle contraction and could cause problems in your cervical spine. When you are working your abs, you need to keep your head leaning forward. Ideally, you should always keep your eyes on your abdomen. The resulting relaxation in the lumbar spine can help you achieve greater flexibility in your vertebrae, which will make curling up easier. Since there is no interference with abdominal contraction, the range of motion is better.

Except for a unilateral exercise like side crunches, you should never lean your head to the side. And if your head is placed to the side, then you must leave it there throughout the exercise. Similarly, shaking your head frenetically when the exercise gets difficult is completely counterproductive. This is when your body should be still.

BREATHING CORRECTLY WHILE DOING ABDOMINAL EXERCISES

You should breathe a specific way during a set of abdominal exercises. The natural tendency is to hold your breath, especially if you are using heavy resistance. Holding your breath will definitely give you strength, but it will also transfer muscle tension from the abdominal muscles to the psoas muscles. In fact, holding your breath makes your abdomen more rigid. Instead of curling up well, the body has a tendency to bend into two segments using the strength of the hip flexor muscles.

Ideally, to work the abdominal muscles, you should exhale very slightly as you curl up using the strength of your rectus abdominis. Emptying your lungs helps you curl your spine to its maximum. In the negative phase, inhale slowly.

Ultimately, intense abdominal exercises interfere with breathing. Breathing occurs only partially. However, you must still try to follow the logic of exhaling during a contraction and inhaling during the negative phase.

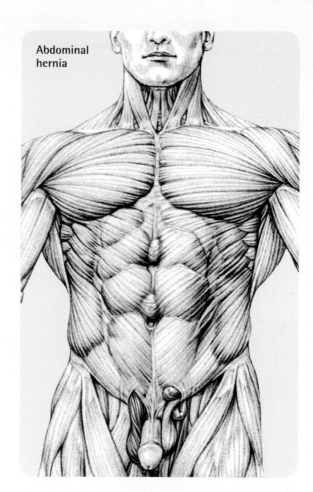

Abdominal hernia

Variations in the morphology of the rectus abdominis

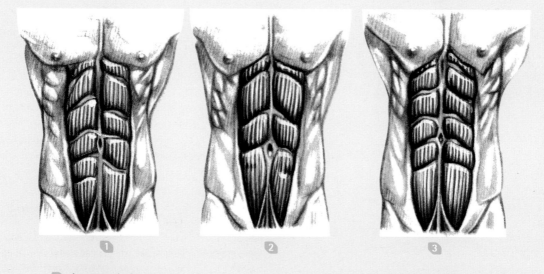

1. Asymmetrical
2. Few tendinous intersections
3. Numerous tendinous intersections

Symmetry is not absolutely necessary in the abs. The appearance of your six-pack can also vary.

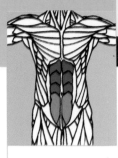

RECTUS ABDOMINIS EXERCISES

1 Crunch

This exercise works the entire abdominal wall but primarily the upper rectus abdominis.

🖐 Lie on your back with your legs bent and your feet on the floor ❶ or your heels resting on a bench ❸. Put your hands behind your head.

🖐 Slowly raise your torso without jerky movements until your shoulders come off the floor ❷. You should curl up and stop as soon as your upper lumbar spine is ready to leave the floor. Pause briefly in this position and contract your abdominal muscles with intensity.

🖐 Slowly return to the starting position and then begin again, always without making any abrupt movements.

- Exhale during the contraction.
- Inhale while lowering your torso to the floor.

ADVANTAGES

The crunch is a simple exercise that works the abdominal muscles without endangering the spine.

DISADVANTAGES

The range of motion in the crunch is rather small (6 inches [15 cm] or so). It is tempting to try to increase it by lifting your entire torso off the floor. The crunch then becomes a sit-up (see page 80). In this case, the abdominal work could become secondary.

RISKS

⚠ If you make any jerky movements with your hands behind your head or with your torso so you can curl up more easily, you run the risk of pinching a disc in your lumbar or cervical spine.

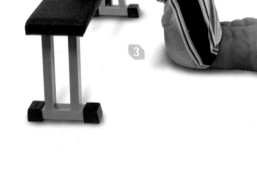

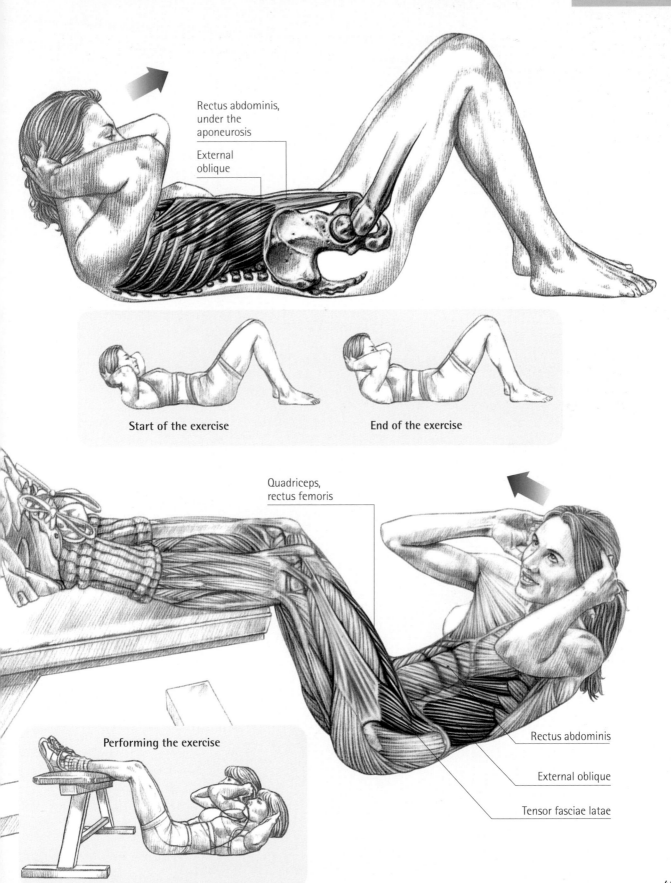

Rectus abdominis, under the aponeurosis

External oblique

Start of the exercise

End of the exercise

Quadriceps, rectus femoris

Rectus abdominis

External oblique

Tensor fasciae latae

Performing the exercise

HELPFUL HINTS

To tone your rectus abdominis, you must continually increase your resistance. The problem with crunches is the lack of resistance. Here are a few strategies to make the exercise more difficult.

1. Stay disciplined.

If you can easily do more than 30 repetitions, then you are likely doing the exercise incorrectly. The most common mistake occurs when you do not deeply contract your abdominal muscles at the top of the movement. The goal is not to do as many repetitions as possible but to contract your abdominal muscles intensely during every repetition. Also, be sure that you are not doing the exercise with momentum or jerky movements from the shoulders and arms. You should do the exercise slowly and correctly, using only your rectus abdominis muscle.

2. Adjust the position of your hands to change the difficulty.

Here are the hand positions from easiest to hardest:

a. Straight arms in front of your body **1** and **2**,

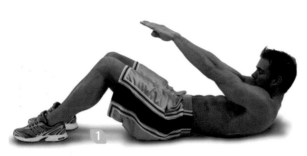

b. Hands on your shoulders **3**,

c. Hands behind your head **4**,

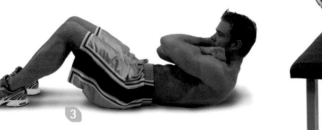

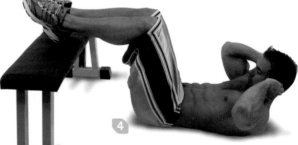

d. Straight arms behind your head **5** and **6**.

An example of a tapering set is to start crunches with straight arms behind you. At failure, bring your hands behind your head, and so on. This will help you get a few more repetitions.

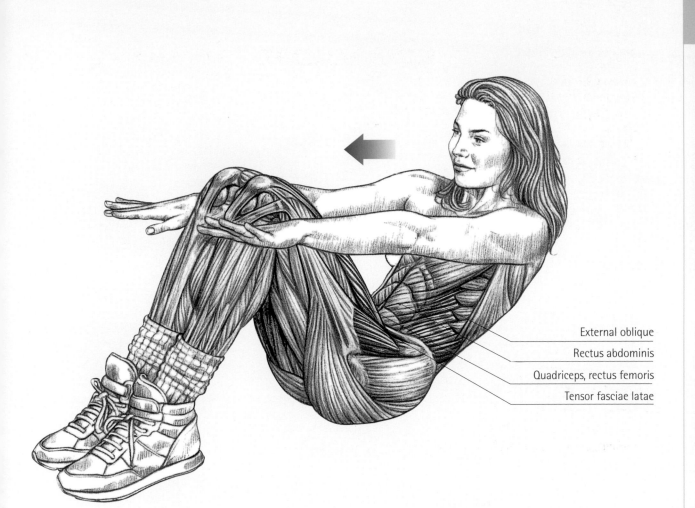

External oblique

Rectus abdominis

Quadriceps, rectus femoris

Tensor fasciae latae

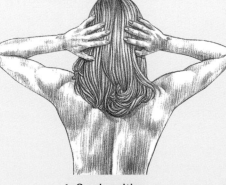

1. Good position

Where to put your hands and elbows

To avoid pulling on your neck, do not clasp your hands behind your head **(2)**. Instead, put them next to each of your ears **(1)**.

Note that the wider apart you hold your elbows, the harder the exercise becomes. Inversely, the closer together and in front your elbows are, the easier the exercise is to do.

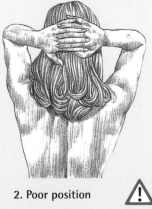

2. Poor position

3. Hold a weight plate behind your head 1 or a dumbbell on your chest 2 to increase the resistance your abdominal muscles must overcome.

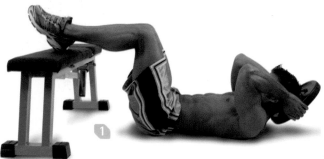

4. Have a partner put a foot on your navel 3.

Start with low resistance, so the foot just brushes your skin. As you work out more, the pressure can increase. A possible tapering set involves backing off the pressure as you get more tired.

5. If you do not have a partner, put a 45-pound (20 kg) weight plate (or several) upright on your abdomen at your navel 4.

If this hurts, place a folded towel between the weight and your belly. In the lengthened position, let the weight really sink into your abdomen. In the contracted position, try to lift the plate as high as possible. At failure, remove the weight and keep going with no weight.

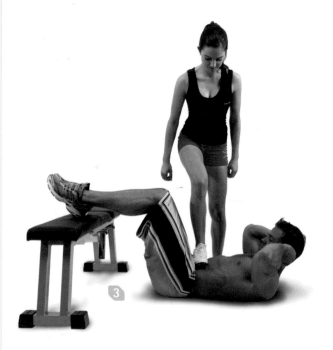

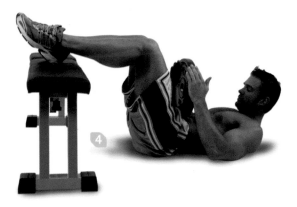

6. Do crunches on a bed, which has two advantages.

First, it is much more comfortable than the floor. Second, the mattress will sink as you raise your torso. This increases your spine's ability to curl up, thereby increasing the contraction of the rectus abdominis.

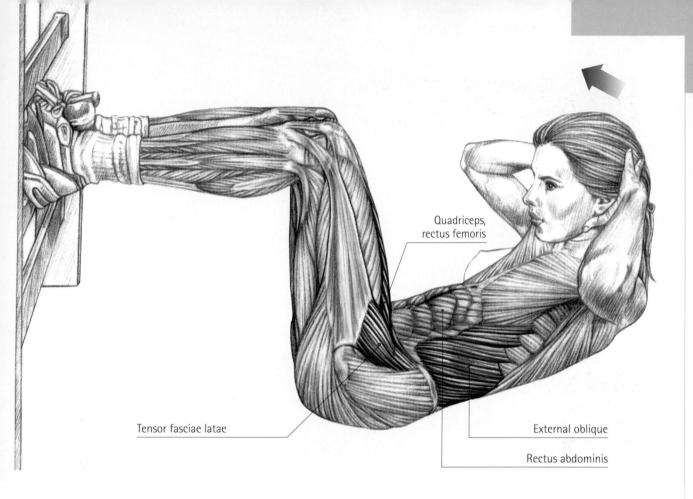

Quadriceps,
rectus femoris

Tensor fasciae latae

External oblique

Rectus abdominis

SHOULD YOU ANCHOR YOUR FEET?

Abdominal exercises like crunches can be done with heavier weights when your feet are held by a partner **1** or pinned under a machine. This increase in strength happens because muscles like the psoas, iliacus, and rectus femoris get involved and take over the work from the abdominal muscles.

If anchoring your feet does not cause you any pain in your low back and lets you better contract your abs, then do not reject the idea. However, if anchoring your feet reduces the work of the rectus abdominis because you are pulling more with your legs (which is often the case), then this is not a good tactic for you.

One tip is to anchor your feet but also let your knees fall to the sides as wide as possible, with your legs bent to a 90-degree angle and the sides of your feet on the floor **2**. This will minimize the involvement of the hip flexor muscles.

The best solution is to begin the exercise with free feet. At failure, anchor your feet so that you can keep going, but you need to be sure that your abs are still contracting as much as possible.

Note: Proportionally, women have lighter torsos and so they have an easier time lifting their torsos without anchoring their feet.

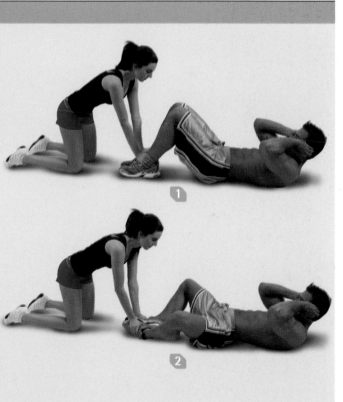

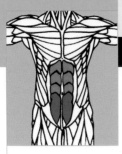

RECTUS ABDOMINIS EXERCISES
2 | Lying Leg Raise

This exercise, also called a reverse crunch, works the entire abdominal wall but targets the lower rectus abdominis in particular.

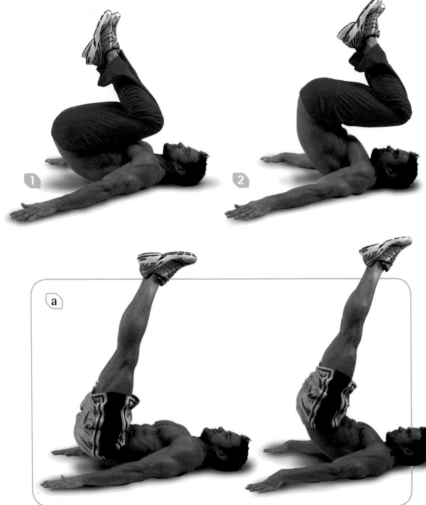

🔵 Lie on your back with your arms on the floor alongside your body and your legs bent to 90 degrees. Lift your buttocks and then your low back by curling up the opposite way you would for a crunch **1**. You must curl up slowly and stop as soon as the upper back starts to come off the floor **2**.

🔵 Try to bring your lower abs toward your chest. The goal is not for them to touch, but by concentrating on that imaginary goal, you will have the right trajectory for the exercise. Pause in the upper position and squeeze your lower abs as hard as you can.

🔵 Slowly lower back to the starting position, stopping before your buttocks touch the floor so that you can maintain continuous tension. Keep your head very straight and do not move your neck.

Variations

a If you keep your legs straight up toward the ceiling, the exercise is easier to do. If you bend your legs so that your calves touch the backs of your thighs, then the exercise will be harder. A good combination is to begin with bent legs. At failure, straighten your legs so that you can get a few more repetitions.

HELPFUL HINT

The goal of this exercise is not so much to lift your legs, but rather to lift your hips. This will indirectly lift the thighs (the thighs always stay in the same position).

Performing the exercise

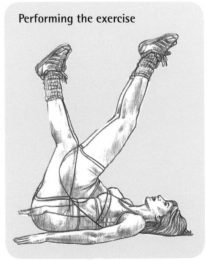

46

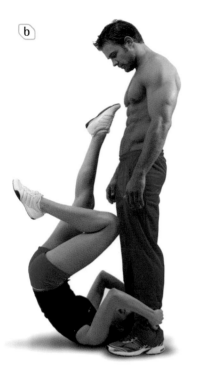

(b)

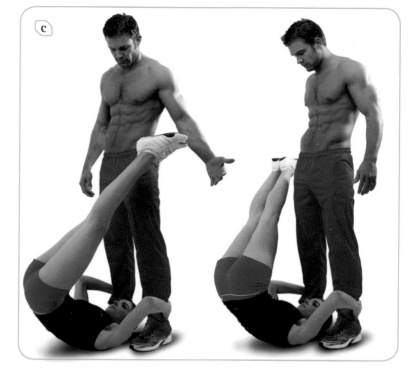

(c)

(b) You can do the exercise one side at a time to make it easier. Since you are moving only one leg at a time, the resistance your abdominal muscles are working against is decreased. You can combine this variation with twisting crunches, which will contract the abs at both ends simultaneously (see figures on page 49).

Warning! This unilateral version is more likely than other versions to harm the spine.

(c) If you rotate your legs to the side, you will target your obliques better.

ADVANTAGES

The lower abdominal muscles are the hardest part of the muscle to target. The lying leg raise is the primary exercise that will teach you to use this lower part.

Of the many variations in leg raises (see part 4), these are the easiest to do because of the low resistance your abdominal muscles have to overcome.

DISADVANTAGES

It is easier to do this exercise incorrectly than it is to do it correctly. A pulling sensation in the low back indicates you are doing the exercise incorrectly. It will take you some time to learn how to really contract the lower part of your abdominal muscles.

RISKS

⚠ If you arch your low back, you are working the wrong muscles and you could be pinching discs in your lumbar spine.

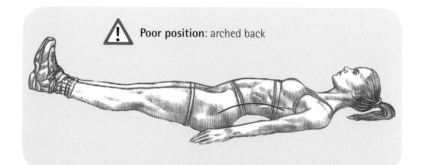

⚠ **Poor position:** arched back

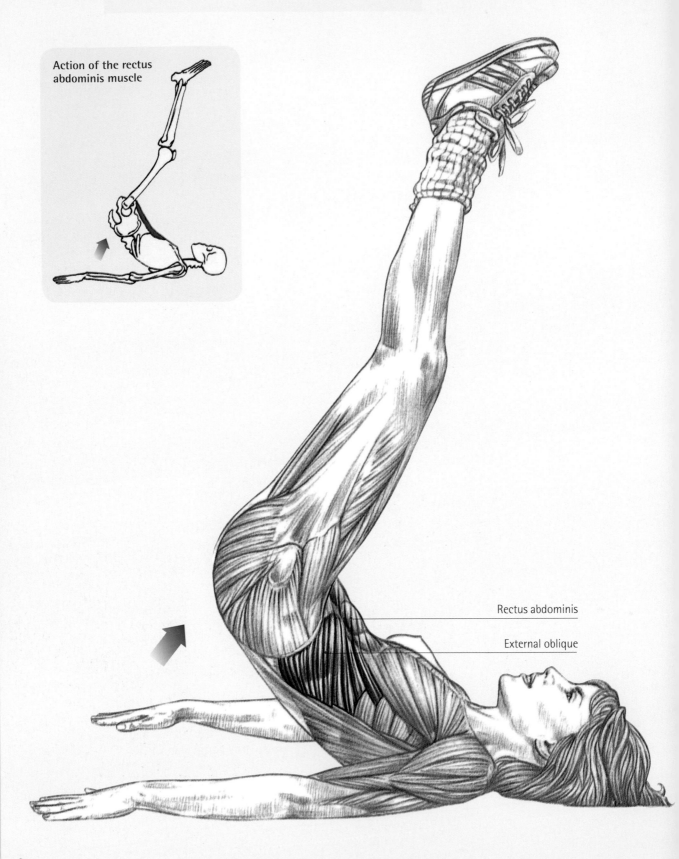

Action of the rectus abdominis muscle

Rectus abdominis

External oblique

Twisting crunch

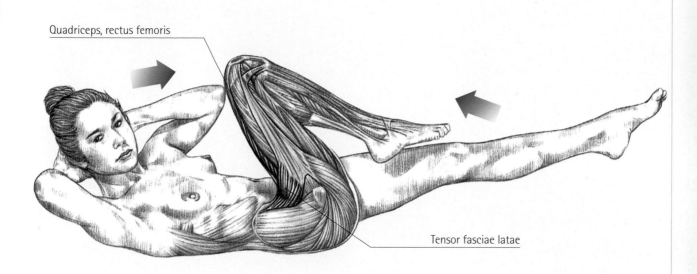

Quadriceps, rectus femoris

Tensor fasciae latae

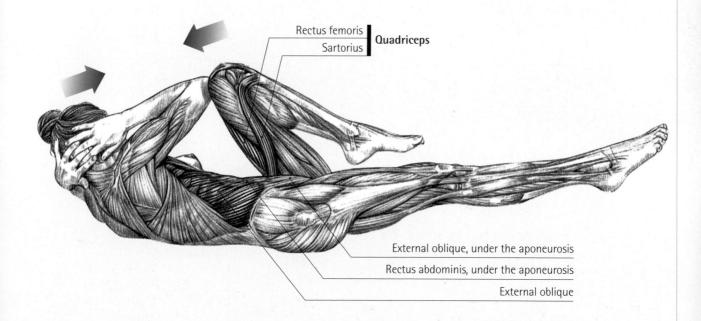

Rectus femoris

Sartorius

Quadriceps

External oblique, under the aponeurosis

Rectus abdominis, under the aponeurosis

External oblique

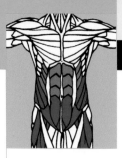

RECTUS ABDOMINIS EXERCISES
3 Seated Leg Raise

This exercise is a variation of the lying leg raise, but it is more difficult to master since there is greater resistance on the abdominal muscles.

🔹 Sit on the edge of a bench, with your arms behind or alongside your body and your hands gripping the edges for stability ❶.

🔹 Bend your legs to 90 degrees and bring your knees toward your chest ❷. The goal is not to touch your knees to your chest, but by concentrating on this imaginary goal, you will get the right trajectory for the exercise. Pause at the highest point of the exercise and squeeze your lower abs tightly.

🔹 Slowly lower your legs back to the starting position, but stop before your thighs are parallel to the floor so that you can maintain continuous tension.

ADVANTAGES

Seated leg raises offer more resistance than lying leg raises. You can use these to continue making progress once the lying-down version has become too easy but leg raises on a pull-up bar are still too hard for you (see page 90).

DISADVANTAGES

When you are sitting down, the weight pressing on your pelvis impedes movement in the spine. It becomes difficult to curve your back to really curl the abdominal muscles from low to high. If you do not curl up well, then the hip flexors, not the abdominal muscles, will perform the exercise.

RISKS

⚠ Avoid arching the low back. Instead, curve it very slightly to reduce pressure on your lumbar discs.

(Variations)

You can alter the resistance of this exercise in these ways:

(a) Straightening your legs more or less (the straighter they are, the more difficult the exercise)

(b) Leaning your torso more or less (the closer it is to parallel to the floor, the easier the exercise)

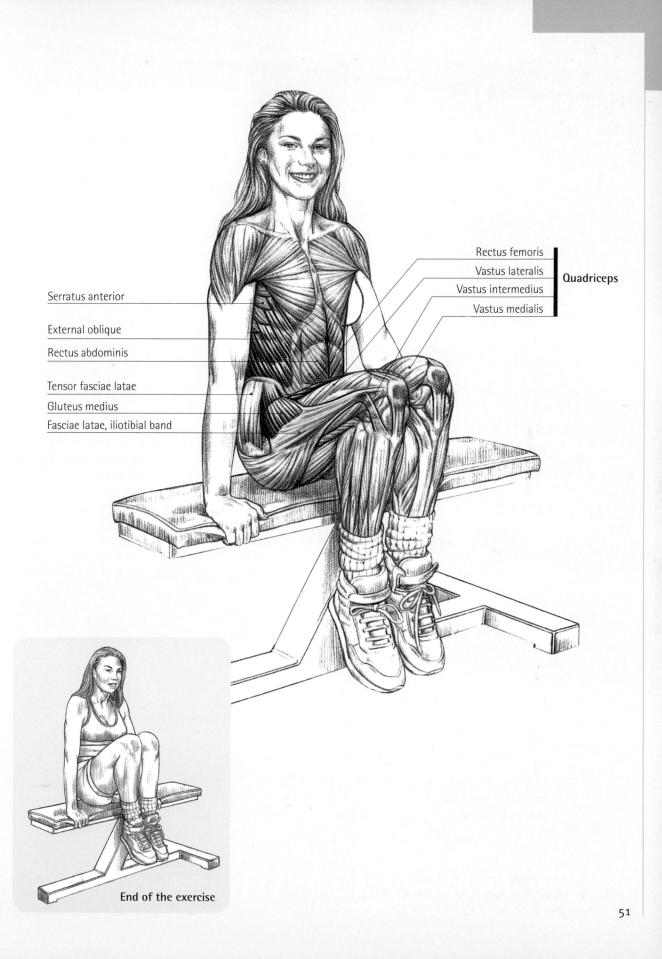

Serratus anterior

External oblique

Rectus abdominis

Tensor fasciae latae

Gluteus medius

Fasciae latae, iliotibial band

Rectus femoris

Vastus lateralis

Vastus intermedius

Vastus medialis

Quadriceps

End of the exercise

51

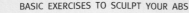

OBLIQUE EXERCISES
Apollo's Belt

DO YOU NEED TO WORK YOUR OBLIQUES?

Unlike the rectus abdominis muscle, which people strive to develop, the obliques are muscles where people prefer definition over bulk. So to eliminate love handles, work with light resistance in long sets rather than with maximum weights.

Greek artists paid special attention to representing the abdominal wall in their statues by highlighting "Apollo's belt." This part of the body is so named because it resembles Apollo's lyre. More precisely, the lower part of the internal oblique muscles forms a junction between the waist and the thighs.

The angle of this junction is more or less oblique at the bottom, as a function of the size and height of the pelvis. If the rectus abdominis reigns over the abdominal muscles, then the internal obliques play a fundamental role in appearance and sex appeal in men. The external obliques do not have great aesthetic value because they make the waist look thick, but the internal obliques give a slender look to the pelvis. Those who admire Greek aestheticism strive to develop the internal obliques.

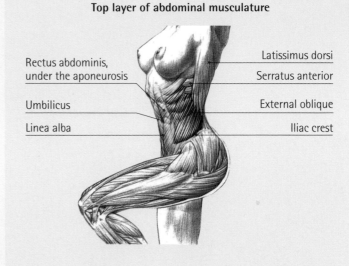

Top layer of abdominal musculature

Rectus abdominis, under the aponeurosis

Umbilicus

Linea alba

Latissimus dorsi

Serratus anterior

External oblique

Iliac crest

Middle layer of abdominal musculature

Costal cartilage

Ribs

Rectus abdominis, under the aponeurosis

Anterior superior iliac spine

Linea alba

Pyramidalis, under the aponeurosis

Pubic symphysis

Pubic tubercule

Internal intercostals

External intercostals

Internal oblique

Iliac crest

Hip bone

Sacrum

Inguinal ligament

Coccyx

Ischiatic spine

Cotyloid cavity, or acetabulum

Ischiatic tuberosity

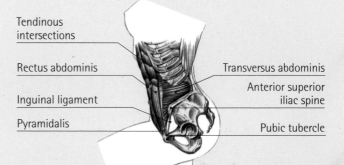

Deep layer of abdominal musculature

Tendinous intersections

Rectus abdominis

Inguinal ligament

Pyramidalis

Transversus abdominis

Anterior superior iliac spine

Pubic tubercle

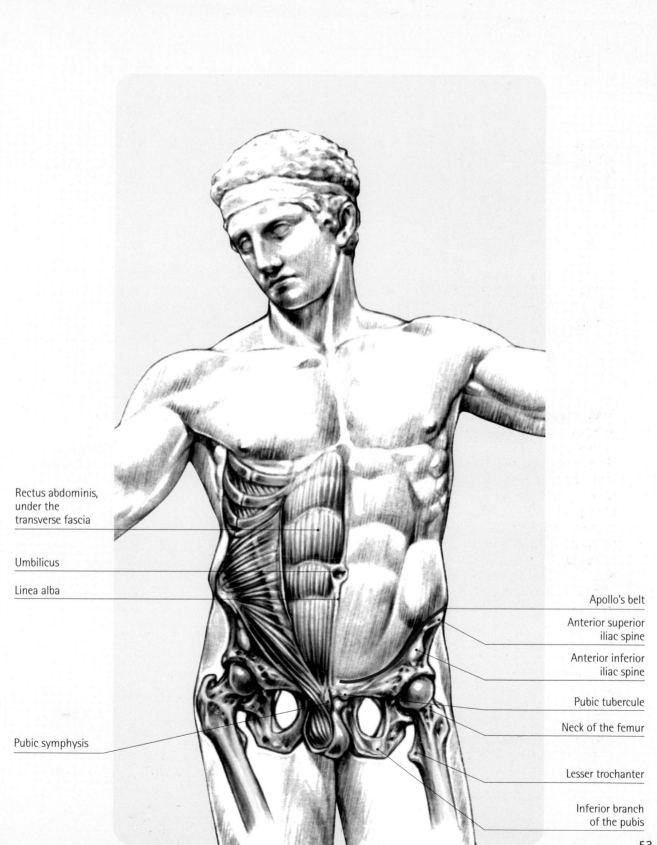

Rectus abdominis, under the transverse fascia

Umbilicus

Linea alba

Pubic symphysis

Apollo's belt

Anterior superior iliac spine

Anterior inferior iliac spine

Pubic tubercule

Neck of the femur

Lesser trochanter

Inferior branch of the pubis

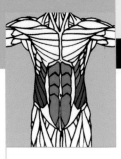

OBLIQUE EXERCISES
1 Twisting Crunch

This exercise targets the obliques as well as the rectus abdominis.

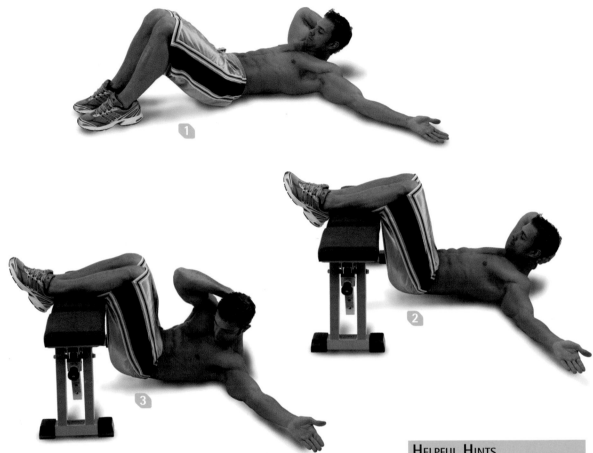

Lie on your back with your legs bent and your feet on the floor **1** or your calves resting on a bench **2**, and your right hand behind your head. Stretch your left arm straight out to your side on the floor so that it serves as a pivot point and accentuates the lateral rotation.

Without jerking, bring your right elbow toward your left thigh using your abdominal muscles **3**. The goal is not to touch your elbow to your thigh; the movement generally ends halfway. But if you concentrate on this imaginary goal, you will have the correct trajectory for the exercise.

Hold the contracted position before lowering your torso. Return slowly to the starting position. To maintain continuous tension, do not rest your head on the floor. Begin again, always without any abrupt movements. Once you have finished this side, repeat the exercise on the other side.

- Exhale during the contraction.
- Inhale while lowering your torso to the floor.

HELPFUL HINTS

You have a couple of options:

- Alternate going to the left for one repetition and then to the right for the next repetition.
- Do all the repetitions in one set to the left, and do all the repetitions in the next set to the right. Note that this left-to-right combination counts as only one set and not two sets.

The position of your hands influences the difficulty of this exercise. Twisting crunches are easier with your arms straight in front of you. You can make the exercise harder by putting one or both of your hands behind your head.

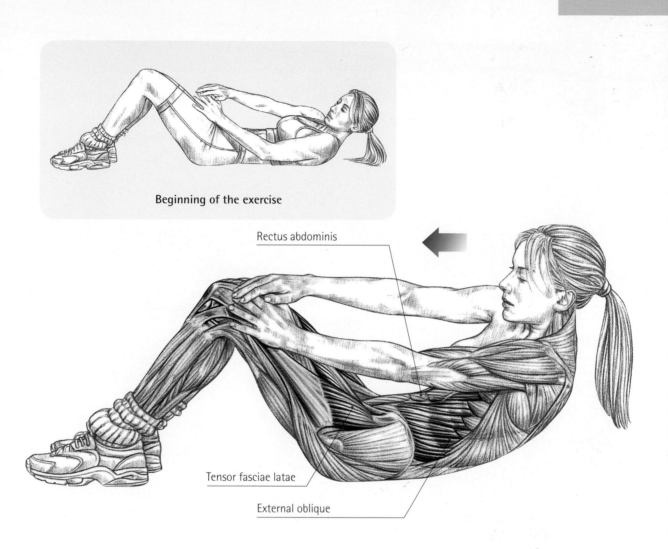

Beginning of the exercise

Rectus abdominis

Tensor fasciae latae

External oblique

Variations

a Arms are straight in front of you with hands toward your knees. Slowly lift your torso without any abrupt movements until your shoulders come off the floor.

b Unlike traditional crunches, bring both hands toward your left knee (see illustration above). Curl up on the side, but stop as soon as the top of your lumbar spine leaves the floor. Pause at the top of the movement and squeeze your abs and obliques tightly.

ADVANTAGES

This is an ideal exercise for circuits or cardio work. While you work the right side, the left side can recover, which lets you do more repetitions without resting your entire body.

DISADVANTAGES

Since you have to work the right side and then the left side, the total length of a set (and your workout) increases.

RISKS

⚠ If you have back pain, the twisting of the spine during this exercise could cause some pain. Lift your torso slowly and do not try to come up too high.

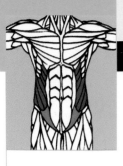

OBLIQUE EXERCISES
2 Side Crunch

This exercise targets the obliques. These muscles support the spine and have an important role in rotating the pelvis, which is crucial for many sports.

🔹 Lie on your left side on the floor. Put your right hand behind your head to support it. Bend your left leg 90 degrees and keep your right leg semibent. The left foot should push gently on the right knee to increase stability ①.

🔹 Using your obliques, bring your right elbow toward your right hip. Your left shoulder will come off the floor a tiny bit ②. Pause at the top of the movement and tightly squeeze your obliques before lowering your torso.

🔹 Bring your left shoulder, but not your head, back to the floor to maintain continuous tension in your obliques. Once you finish a set on the right, move on to the left side.

HELPFUL HINT

The trajectory of this exercise is not straight. Instead, the torso rotates slightly from back to front to contract the obliques tightly.

Variations

a The placement of your free arm determines the degree of resistance for the exercise. We have described an intermediate position with your hand behind your head. By stretching your free arm above your head (in line with your body), you increase the resistance your obliques have to overcome.

b You can decrease the resistance by stretching your arm toward your thigh, always keeping it in line with your body. Here is a good combination:

- Begin the exercise with your arm above your head.
- At failure, put your hand behind your head to get a few more repetitions.
- When you reach failure again, stretch your arm toward your legs so you can continue the exercise.
- When you are worn out, do a few forced repetitions by grabbing the back of your thigh with your hand. Use your arm to help pull your torso and reduce the workload on the obliques. This technique to increase intensity is known as tapering, and it quickly tires out the obliques and reduces the number of sets that you need to do.

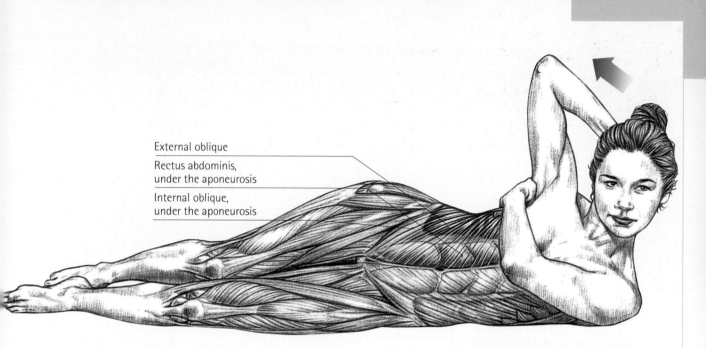

External oblique

Rectus abdominis, under the aponeurosis

Internal oblique, under the aponeurosis

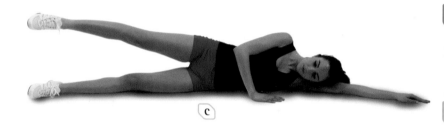

c

c Instead of moving your torso, you can lift your thigh while your legs are straight and in line with your torso. Be careful not to lift above 45 degrees so that you can really concentrate your efforts in the obliques and not the buttocks.

d

d You can also lift your torso and leg simultaneously from this initial position.

NOTE

It is better to end your core workout with obliques rather then begin it with side crunches. The abs, not the obliques, are your priority.

TIP

Place one hand on the obliques that are working so that you will be better able to feel their contraction.

ADVANTAGES

This exercise targets the obliques perfectly. You can feel the muscles working immediately, as long as you are in the correct position.

DISADVANTAGES

Except for strength sports, you should be careful not to overwork your obliques. These muscles make the waist bigger, which is not the look you are after. Instead, use long sets with light resistance so you can accentuate the muscle definition and burn fat around the waist.

RISKS

⚠ Do not make any abrupt movements with your head to get a few more repetitions, because your cervical spine is in a vulnerable position when your head is held up in the air.

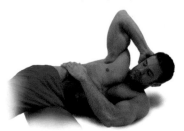

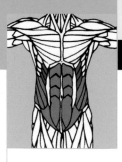

STABILITY EXERCISES
1 Static Stability, Back Against Wall

This static exercise works the transversus abdominis and the obliques as well as numerous deep muscles that support the spine.

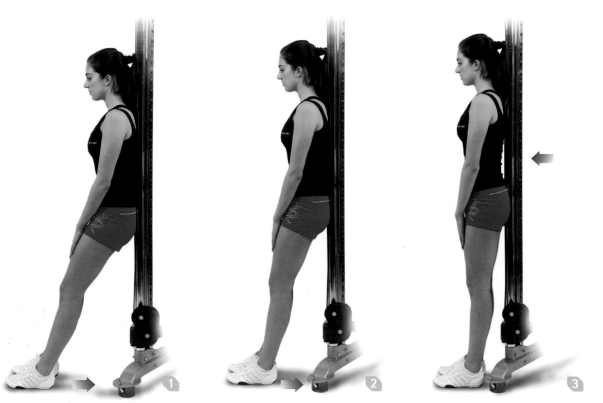

🔵 Stand with your back against a wall. Your spine should be touching the wall. To do this, move your feet forward about 20 inches (50 cm) and keep your legs straight **1**.

🔵 Little by little, bring your feet closer to the wall and strive to avoid arching your lumbar spine. Rather, you should press your low back into the wall as much as possible **2**.

🔵 When you feel your lumbar spine coming off the wall, you should stop moving your feet **3**.

Hold the isometric contraction for as long as possible (at least 15 seconds).

HELPFUL HINT

Even though this exercise might seem easy, you will feel quite a few abdominal muscles contracting. Since these muscles are not used to working like this, you will notice that they get tired relatively quickly.

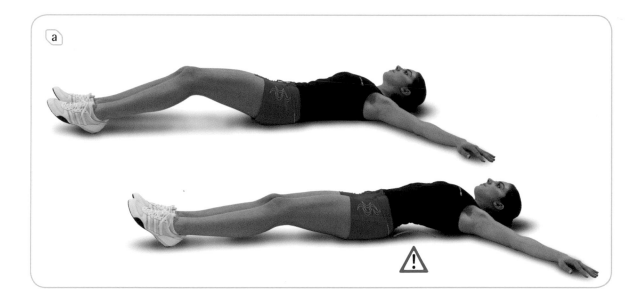

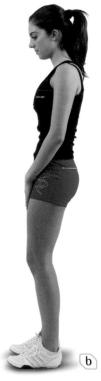

(Variations)

a If you cannot hold the standing position for 15 seconds, then do this same exercise while lying on the floor with your legs bent to 90 degrees. Stretch your legs out gently without arching your back. The goal here is to press your low back into the floor as much as possible, as if you were trying to push through the floor. Try not to push on your heels too much while doing this, though.

When you feel that your lumbar spine is coming off of the floor, stop straightening your legs.

b When the exercise against a wall becomes too easy, try to do it standing up without leaning against a wall.

ADVANTAGES

Performing this exercise regularly will help prevent back pain by recruiting numerous muscles that support the lumbar spine.

DISADVANTAGES

Because this is not an impressive exercise, many people neglect to do it.

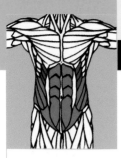

STABILITY EXERCISES
2 Plank

This exercise works the entire abdominal wall statically.

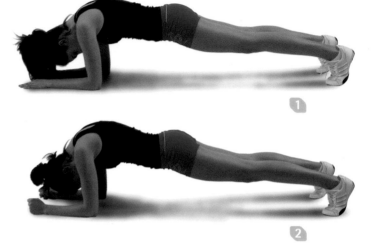

🔹 Stretch out facedown on the floor, and support your weight on your forearms and toes **1**. Hold this static position for at least 15 seconds while keeping your body as straight as possible.

🔹 If the weight of your head becomes too uncomfortable, bend your neck forward **2**.

A yoga mat (or at least a towel) will help prevent unnecessary pain in your forearms.

Variations

a To increase the difficulty of this exercise, a partner can place a weight plate on your back or sit on you. In this case, be very careful not to arch your back.

b You can work the obliques if you do this same exercise in a side position. If this variation is too difficult at first, use your free hand for support by placing it on the floor in front of you.

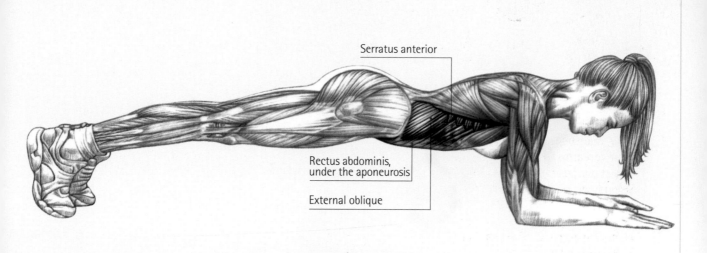

Serratus anterior

Rectus abdominis,
under the aponeurosis

External oblique

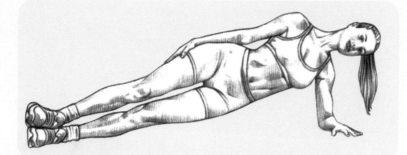

ADVANTAGES

This stabilization exercise requires no equipment and can be done in very little time. You and your friends could make this into a friendly competition by seeing who can hold the position the longest!

DISADVANTAGES

Static work is not the best form of exercise to improve the appearance of your abdominal muscles. However, this strengthening exercise is perfect for athletes who want muscular stability for defense (combat sports or team contact sports).

HELPFUL HINT

If you have trouble putting your palms on the floor, make fists and put your hands in a neutral position (with only the pinkies touching the floor).

RISKS

⚠ If you arch your back, you could pinch your discs. Even though holding your breath will make this exercise easier, you should not do it! If you feel like your breathing is affected, exhale with tiny breaths.

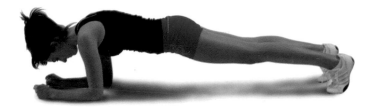

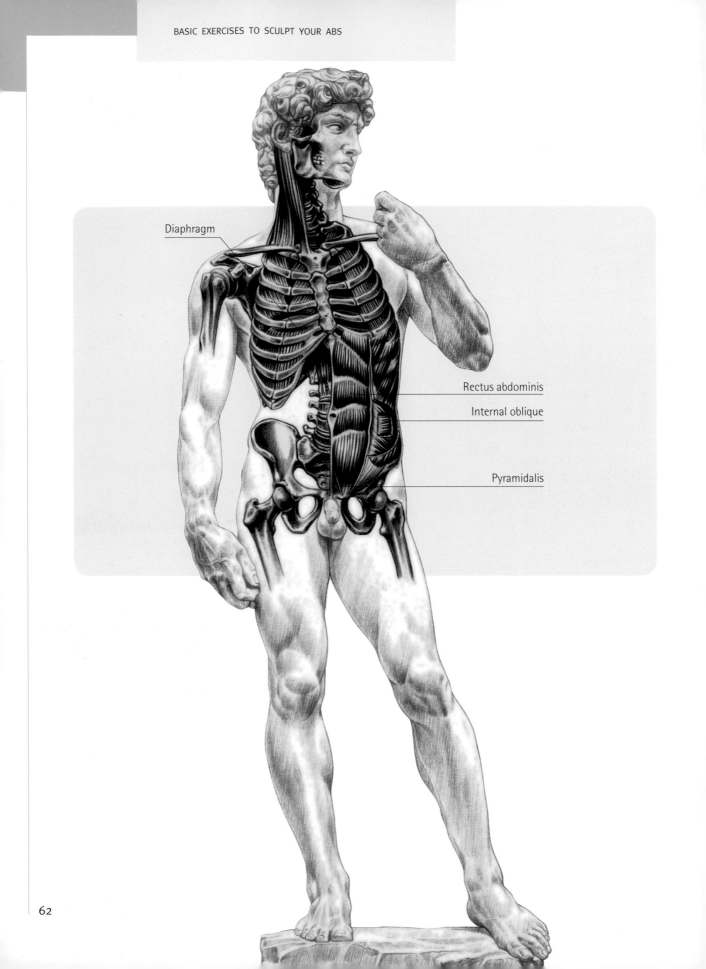

Diaphragm

Rectus abdominis

Internal oblique

Pyramidalis

1 Lying Rib Cage Expansion With a Weight

By making the expansion of the rib cage more difficult, this exercise strengthens the muscles used for inhalation.

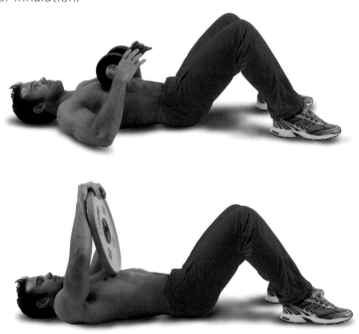

ENDURANCE AND THE MUSCLES USED FOR BREATHING

Scientific research has shown that during an endurance activity, the muscles used for breathing, especially the diaphragm, get tired. As with other muscles, this fatigue decreases performance. Diaphragm exercises also profoundly improve endurance. Athletes who have trained in this manner also have bigger diaphragms than sedentary people. Breathing exercises will help alleviate shortness of breath during prolonged athletic effort.

🖐 Lie on your back and put a dumbbell or weight plate on your chest. Inhale deeply so that you expand your rib cage to its maximum, and then exhale to contract your rib cage.

Variation

You can use a resistance band to squeeze your chest lightly during endurance activities. This will make it harder to expand your rib cage and will help strengthen the muscles used for breathing.

HELPFUL HINT

This exercise will do nothing for your endurance unless you do it in long sets (at least 50 repetitions).

RISKS

⚠ Do not begin with a heavy weight that will crush your ribs. Start with a light weight to get your rib cage used to this exercise.

63

BREATHING EXERCISES TO IMPROVE ATHLETIC PERFORMANCE

2 Diaphragm Contraction

This exercise targets the diaphragm and the muscles responsible for breathing.

🔲 Get on the floor on all fours and pull in your belly as much as you can while inhaling ❶ and ❷. Relax your muscles when you exhale.

Variations

a If you have trouble doing this exercise, practice it sitting up or kneeling (which are a little bit easier). You can also use your arms to help you.

b You can also lie on your back (which is much easier).

c To get the maximum benefits for endurance, you can try this combination:

- Begin on all fours until your breathing muscles are fatigued.
- When fatigued, turn over on your back so you can continue the exercise using the easier version.

NOTE

This exercise is extremely easy . . . at first. After 20 repetitions, you will feel an unusual fatigue. This is when your breathing muscles begin to get stronger. Do as many repetitions as you can!

ADVANTAGES

This exercise also works the transversus abdominis, which is the muscle that gives you a flat abdomen.

RISKS

⚠ Hyperventilation could cause a slight passing dizzy spell.

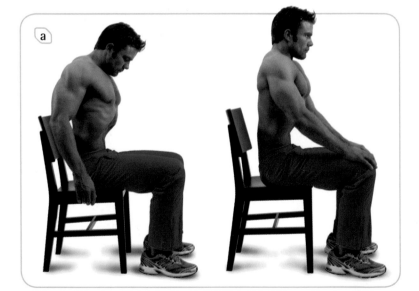

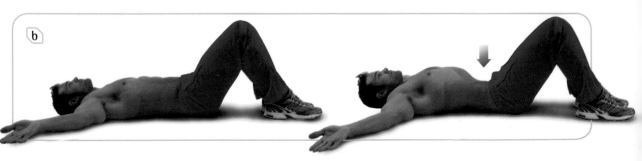

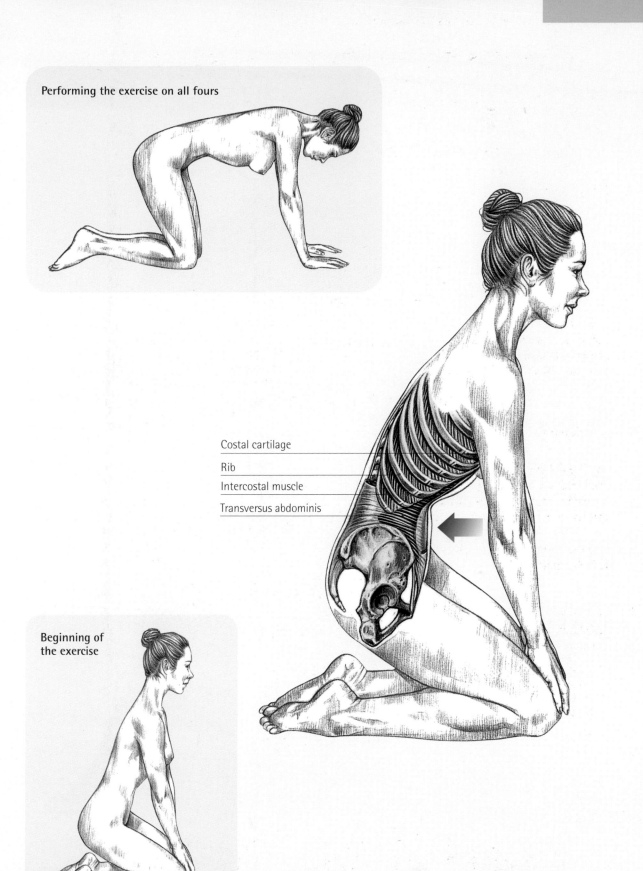

Performing the exercise on all fours

Costal cartilage

Rib

Intercostal muscle

Transversus abdominis

Beginning of the exercise

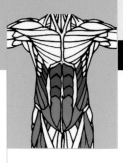

STRETCHING THE ABDOMINAL MUSCLES
1 On a Stability Ball

This exercise stretches the abdominal muscles and relaxes the back.

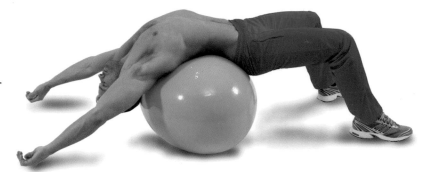

 Lie on your back on a stability ball with your legs bent to 90 degrees and your feet firmly on the floor for stability. Put your arms straight up and keep them in line with your head. Lower your buttocks toward the floor while stretching your arms as far away as possible.

Take 30 seconds to 1 minute to stretch your abdominal muscles thoroughly.

ADVANTAGES

You can stretch your abdominal muscles while your spine is perfectly supported.

DISADVANTAGES

To keep your belly very flat, do not stretch your abdominal muscles too often. Do not overdo this exercise, neither in quantity nor in range of motion.

RISKS

⚠ If you suffer from back pain, you need to discuss any abdominal stretching with your doctor.

Variation

With bent arms

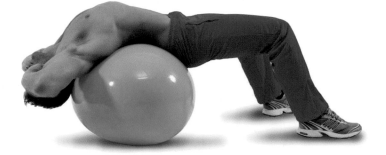

STRETCHING THE HIP FLEXORS

As you arch your back, you artificially push your belly forward. Overstrengthening the psoas and iliac muscles causes the belly to push too far forward this way. It is important to work on flexibility in your hip flexors to minimize arching the back. These stretches will quickly help you lose inches off your waist and minimize the risk of pinching a disc.

Tilting of the Pelvis

The pelvis generally tilts a bit more forward in women than in men. This forward tilt makes the buttocks stick out while the pubic bone is tucked in between the thighs. This creates the impression that the lower abdomen sticks out slightly. This typically feminine little tummy contrasts with the vertical abdominal wall that is more frequently found in men (because a typical male pelvis does not tilt forward as much).

This special positioning of the female pelvis protects women when they are pregnant. It ensures that the infant does not compromise the viscera too much since the abdominal wall supports a portion of the infant's weight.

Abdominal–Lumbar Balance

It is important to work both the abdominal muscles and the erector spinae muscles equally.

Underworking or overworking one of these two muscle groups can cause poor posture, which, in the long run, can lead to other problems.

Example: If the lower part of the erector spinae muscles (sacrolumbar mass) is too strong and the abdominal muscles are too weak, it can lead to hyperlordosis with an abdominal ptosis. This posture issue, if it is caught in time, can sometimes be corrected by doing abdominal strengthening exercises.

Conversely, abdominal muscles that are too strong combined with weakened erector spinae muscles, particularly in the upper back (spinalis dorsi, longissimus dorsi, and iliocostalis dorsi), can lead to kyphosis (rounding of the upper back) and a loss of the lumbar curve. This posture issue can be corrected by doing specific exercises to strengthen the erector spinae muscles.

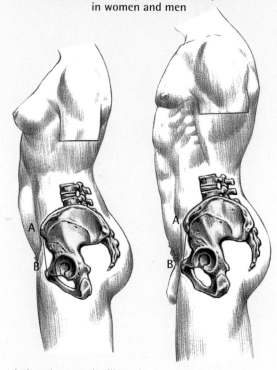

Comparison of the position of the pelvis
in women and men

A: Anterior–superior iliac spine
B: Pubic tubercule

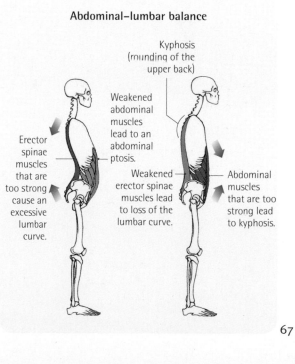

Abdominal–lumbar balance

Kyphosis (rounding of the upper back)

Erector spinae muscles that are too strong cause an excessive lumbar curve.

Weakened abdominal muscles lead to an abdominal ptosis.

Weakened erector spinae muscles lead to loss of the lumbar curve.

Abdominal muscles that are too strong lead to kyphosis.

STRETCHING THE HIP FLEXORS
1 Lunge

This exercise stretches the hip flexors when it is done with a very upright torso.

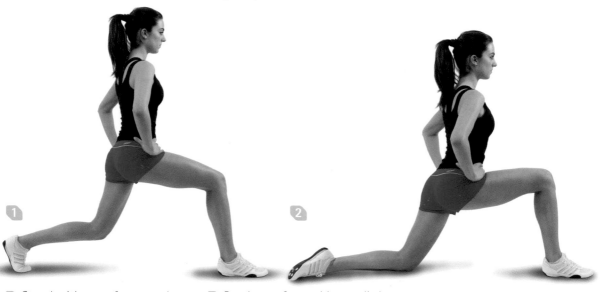

🖐 Stand with your feet together and legs straight. Put your hands on your hips or your thighs. If you have balance problems, hold on to a wall or a chair. Begin the exercise by taking one step forward with your right leg ❶. If you're a beginner, you can bend the left leg a bit. If you are more advanced, keep the left leg straight to make the exercise harder.

🖐 Bend your forward knee a little bit farther ❷. If you're a beginner, lower yourself no more than 8 inches [20 cm]; if advanced, you can go farther, even resting your back knee on the ground. Hold the position for 30 seconds to 1 minute to stretch the hip flexors well.

Repeat the same exercise on the left leg.

ADVANTAGES
Lunges are an excellent way to stretch all the muscles in the lower limbs.

DISADVANTAGES
It might be tempting to lean your torso forward to make the stretch easier. Instead, it is better to take a smaller step forward so you can keep your torso upright.

RISKS
⚠ Lunges stretch the psoas muscles, and this has a tendency to arch your low back if you are not very flexible.

NOTE
As the stretch in the hip flexors increases, you will notice that
- the back leg is straighter,
- the step forward is larger, and
- the torso remains upright.

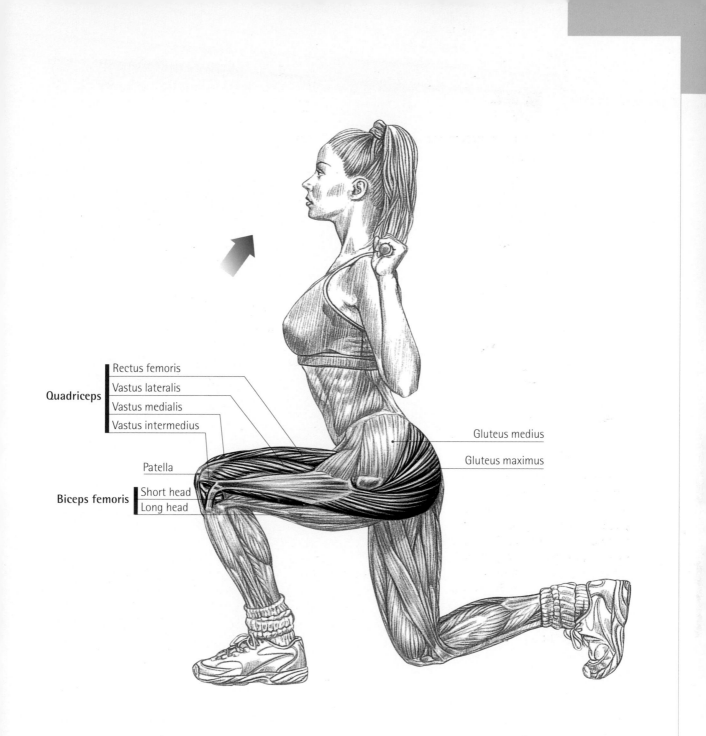

Quadriceps
- Rectus femoris
- Vastus lateralis
- Vastus medialis
- Vastus intermedius

Patella

Biceps femoris
- Short head
- Long head

Gluteus medius

Gluteus maximus

STRETCHING THE LOW BACK

Spinal cord

Nucleus pulposus

Annulus fibrosus

Vertebral body

Spinous process

Articular process

Spinal canal

As the spine moves, a disc is pinched in the front and bulges in the back. The fluid in the nucleus pulposus migrates toward the back and can eventually compress the nerves, resulting in sciatica.

All of your daily activities compromise the health of your spine. The low back (lumbar region) is the part used most often. Because of the weight pressing on the intervertebral discs, the fluid enclosed in the discs is squeezed out. But this fluid is vital to the health of the spine because it absorbs shock. This explains why you are about 0.5 to 1 inch (~1.3-2.5 cm) shorter in the evening than in the morning. When the discs are dehydrated, the back is more vulnerable and unstable, which increases the risk of injury and pain.

When you lie down to sleep, the pressure on the spine decreases and the discs fill up with fluid again.

However, you might stay very stiff throughout the night because of overactive muscles. Not only might you sleep poorly, but the pressure on the spine does not decrease. You might wake up feeling tired and have persistent backaches.

Intervertebral disc

Transverse process

Vertebral body

Articular process

Spinous process

Intervertebral foramen (where a nerve from the spinal cord passes through)

Vertebrae

1. Compressed   2. Not compressed

Annulus fibrosus

Nucleus pulposus

Vertebral body

Preventing Low Back Pain

Doing abdominal and core exercises relaxes the lumbar region, and you can use these exercises to stretch and relieve pain in the low back. At night, this spinal relaxation will help you sleep better and will promote healing in the low back. Here are two preventive exercises that you can do.

Deep muscles of the back

Vertebra

Iliocostalis cervicis

Longissimus cervicis

Rib

Iliocostalis dorsi

Longissimus dorsi

Spinalis dorsi

Iliocostalis lumborum

Quadratus lumborum

Aponeurosis

Semispinalis capitis

Splenius capitis

Splenius cervicis

Serratus posterior superior

Serratus posterior inferior

Hip bone

Sacrum

Coccyx

Femur

1 Relaxation Stretch on a Stability Ball

This exercise relaxes the back and abdominal muscles and promotes decompression in the spine.

Version 1

Lie flat on your front on a stability ball with your legs bent, toes on the floor, and arms hanging loosely. Relax your whole body for 30 seconds to 1 minute while supported by the ball in order to decompress your back 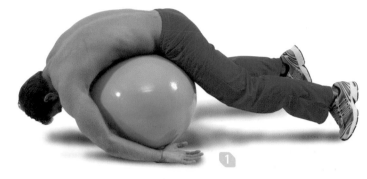 to 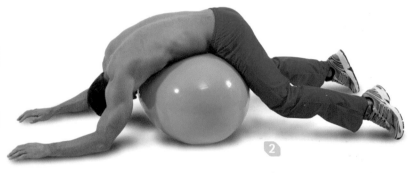.

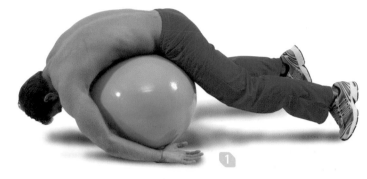

ADVANTAGES

These exercises will encourage you to release tension in your back.

DISADVANTAGES

You need a stability ball to do this exercise.

RISKS

⚠ If you suffer from back pain, you need to discuss any back stretches with your doctor.

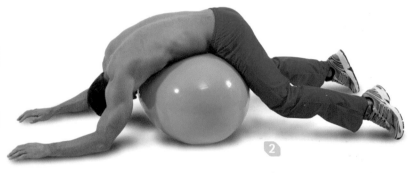

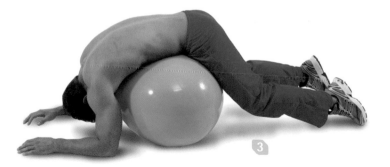

Version 2

Lie on your back on a stability ball with your legs bent and your feet flat on the floor for stability. Put your arms straight out in line with your head. Lower your buttocks to the floor while stretching your arms as far away as you can 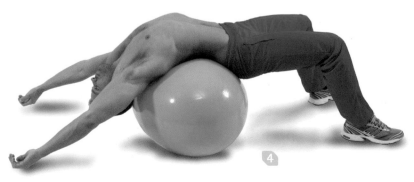. Hold this position to relax the spine and abdominal muscles.

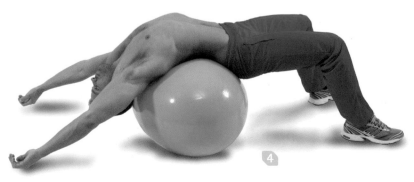

STRETCHES FOR THE LOW BACK
2 Hanging From a Pull-Up Bar

This static relaxation exercise stretches the back,
which promotes decompression in the lumbar spine.

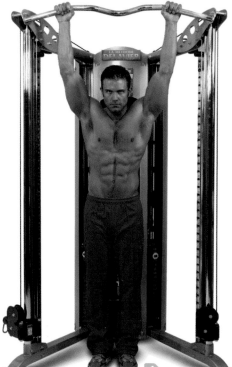

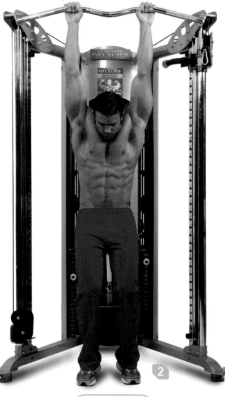

Grab a pull-up bar with your hands shoulder-width apart using an overhand grip (thumbs facing each other) **1**.

ADVANTAGES

When you are suspended, you are mimicking nocturnal decompression. The recovery of your spine will be better, and you will sleep better too.

DISADVANTAGES

This exercise requires a pull-up bar.

RISKS

⚠ If you suffer from back pain, you need to discuss any lumbar stretching with your doctor.

The weight of your body rests on your legs, so transfer it slowly to your arms while relaxing your back **2**. Take 30 seconds to release the tension in your lumbar spine completely. Once you are done with the stretch, transfer the weight of your body back to your legs and slowly let go of the bar.

HELPFUL HINTS

The spine should lengthen freely. If, however, it stays compressed, this means your lumbar muscles are tight. You need to relax them, which is something you will learn to do with time.

To help them relax, first do a set of abdominal exercises, and then move immediately to hanging from the pull-up bar. The resulting temporary fatigue will help relax the muscles that support the spine.

Variations

If you take on too much weight with your hands, you will create a reflex contraction in the back. This will make it difficult to relax your spine. At first, it is better to transfer only a portion of your body weight to your arms by brushing the floor with

a your toes (calves facing behind you) or

b your heels (your legs stay in front of you).

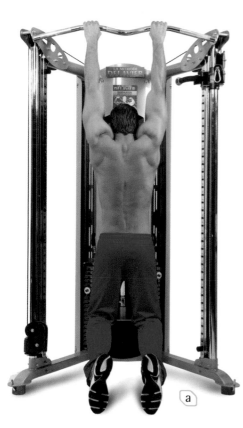

a

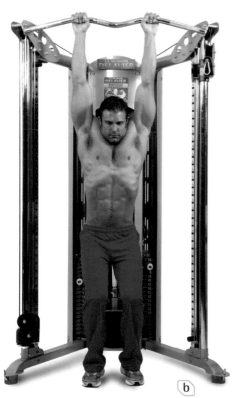

b

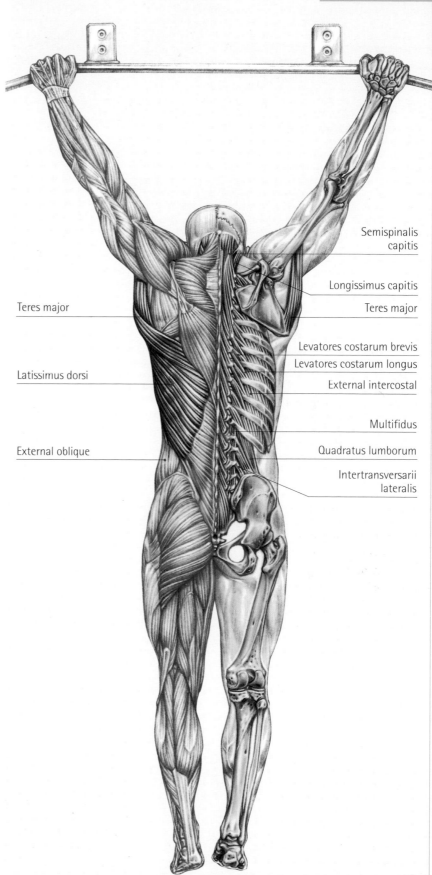

Semispinalis capitis

Longissimus capitis

Teres major

Levatores costarum brevis

Levatores costarum longus

External intercostal

Multifidus

Quadratus lumborum

Intertransversarii lateralis

Teres major

Latissimus dorsi

External oblique

PART 4

Advanced Exercises and Techniques

Three Difficulties of Abdominal Work

The first improvements to the abdominal wall are relatively easy to achieve if you are following a good program. But beyond this golden period, which lasts a few months, the abs become more and more resistant to progress. It is a good idea to formulate more sophisticated training strategies so you can continue to improve your abs.

Here are three main difficulties affecting the abdominal wall:

1. The lower abs are not as strong as the upper abs.
2. A six-pack is not developed enough.
3. A lack of tone in the abdominal wall gives you a large belly.

How to Isolate Upper Abdominal Work From Lower Abdominal Work

Is it possible to isolate upper abdominal work from lower abdominal work? Does the rectus abdominis contract over its entire length? Or does it contract at the top or the bottom? Is it a waste of time to want to work the lower abs in addition to the upper abs? The truth is that for many people the upper abs are better developed than the lower part. The six-pack may look good at the top, but the curve at the lower part looks more like a beer belly! If the rectus abdominis worked equally hard at both ends, this disparity would not exist.

Medical studies show that the rectus abdominis contracts in segments. This segmentation is explained by the fact that the upper part of the muscle and the lower part of the muscle are innervated separately. Exercises in which you lift your torso mostly work the upper part (but not exclusively). Exercises where you lift your pelvis target the lower part better.

Since it is harder to strengthen the lower abs than the upper abs, the lower part requires special attention.

Conclusion

The abdominal muscles work at both the top and bottom. Advanced ab training should make the lower part a priority because the lower part

- is the hardest to develop,
- supports the spine better,
- prevents bloating, and
- is more likely to have fat stored there.

Why Are the Lower Abdominal Muscles So Hard to Develop?

It is rare to see abs perfectly developed along their entire length. There are several reasons for this classic delay in developing the bottom part of the abs.

1. It is difficult to recruit that part of the muscle.

A lack of activity does not encourage the lower region to get involved in abdominal exercises. The central nervous system more readily recruits the upper part, which explains why it is possible to do a leg lift using your upper abdominals when it is the lower part that should be initiating the movement.

2. Lower abs lack strength.

Since the lower abdominal muscles are not very bulky, they are weak even though we often ask them to lift the entire weight of the thighs. To alleviate this inadequacy between the weight and their strength, the brain mobilizes the powerful hip flexors (psoas and iliac muscles), which can easily substitute for the lower abs.

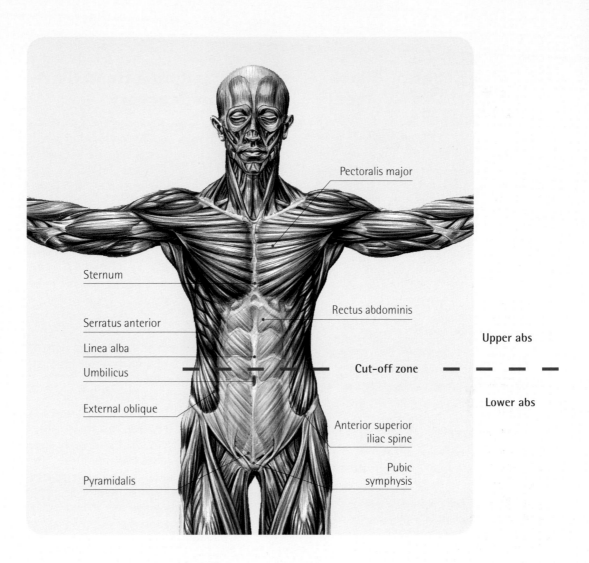

Pectoralis major

Sternum

Serratus anterior

Linea alba

Umbilicus

External oblique

Pyramidalis

Rectus abdominis

Cut-off zone

Anterior superior
iliac spine

Pubic
symphysis

Upper abs

Lower abs

3. It is difficult to isolate the lower part.

Perfectly isolating the lower abs is difficult, especially when the weight increases. For this reason, leg lifts are technically much more complex to master than crunches.

4. Lower abs are not robust.

Since they are not used very often, the lower abdominal muscles are not very resistant to fatigue, and they cannot handle a heavy amount of training.

5. Many exercises are inappropriate.

Exercises that are known for working the lower abs are generally inappropriate. The purpose of the lower part of the rectus abdominis is to lift your buttocks off the floor when you are lying down. Its role is not to lift the thighs and even less so to do leg flutters.

Three Zones of Attack for Total Development

The abdominal wall should be trained in three distinct areas:

1. Lower abs
2. Upper abs
3. Muscles responsible for torso rotation

Avoid the classic mistake of doing crunches for your upper abs and ignoring the other two zones. Though you do not need to work all three zones in the same workout, you should be careful not to neglect any of the three zones.

Relative Importance of Each Zone

These three zones are not of equal importance. The most important zone, and therefore the most problematic, is the lower part of the abdominal muscles. If you are concerned about your appearance, then it is reasonable to rank the three zones this way:

- 50 percent lower abdominal work
- 30 percent upper abdominal work
- 20 percent exercises involving rotation

For example, if your workout consists of 10 sets of abdominal and core exercises and you are exercising twice a week, you should do the following:

- 10 sets for your lower abs
- 6 sets for your upper abs
- 4 sets involving rotation

This distribution provides a good base for your workout. But you can adjust the importance of each zone based on your individual needs. For example, if you are trying to get rid of your love handles or if your favorite sport involves a lot of rotation, then doing rotation exercises will be the most important for you. In this case, you could rank the sets this way:

- 10 sets involving rotation
- 6 sets for your lower abs
- 4 sets for your upper abs

Getting a Head Start on Recovery

Getting a head start on recovery is a strategy that allows you to work your abdominal and core muscles again productively even if they are not yet fully recovered from a previous workout. This partial-recovery approach allows you to increase the frequency of your core workouts while avoiding overtraining. This strategy is intended only for experienced athletes who are looking for fast results.

In this method, you select a single abdominal exercise per workout and alternate your choices for every workout. Choosing a single exercise has many benefits, especially for recovery. By alternating exercises from one workout to the next, you give the different nerve pathways more recovery time. In fact, for advanced athletes, we recommend that you avoiding "frying" your neuromuscular pathways—that is, avoid always doing the same exercises.

For example, during the first workout, do only lying leg raises for the lower abs. The next workout, do only crunches for the upper abs. Then repeat the cycle. The advantage here is that the neuromuscular circuit used for lying leg raises does not need to be 100 percent recovered in order for you to be able to do crunches. However, it is essential that the neuromuscular unit be fully recovered before you do lying leg raises again. By constantly rotating your exercises, you can space your core workouts more closely together even though your central nervous system is only partially recovered. But, if you do lying leg raises and crunches in the same workout, you must wait for both of these neuromuscular circuits to fully recover before you can exercise your abdominal and core muscles again.

So, our sample workout with priority placed on the lower abs involves the following:

- The first workout in week 1 will include 10 sets of exercises for the lower abs.
- The second workout in week 1 will include 6 sets for the upper abs and 4 sets of rotation exercises.
- In week 2, you will repeat the cycle.

1 Double Crunch

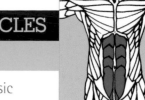

This exercise isolates the entire rectus abdominis. Unlike the classic crunch, which primarily works the upper part, the double crunch works the upper and lower abs at the same time.

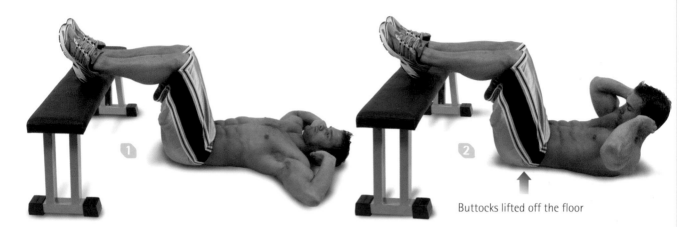

Buttocks lifted off the floor

⬤ Lie on your back with your legs bent to 90 degrees and your heels resting on a bench ❶.

⬤ Simultaneously lift your shoulders and your buttocks ❷. Curl up by bringing your hips and shoulders closer together. Stop as soon as your shoulders and lumbar spine have left the floor. Pause in this position and tightly squeeze your abdominal muscles.

⬤ Return to the starting position slowly and then begin again, always without any abrupt movements.

- Exhale during the contraction.
- Inhale as you lower your torso to the floor.

ADVANTAGES

The abdominal work is more complete in this exercise than in classic crunches, because the head and the pelvis come closer together at the same time. This shortens the muscle at both ends.

DISADVANTAGES

Even though this exercise looks easy, mastering it is not. You can easily do this exercise with the wrong muscles, which is counterproductive to the goal of strengthening your abdominal muscles.

HELPFUL HINTS

Because you are lifting your buttocks, you will not be able to raise your torso as high as you can with classic crunches. Only the shoulders, not the whole upper back, should leave the floor. However, you should lift your buttocks as high as possible.

Because it is easier, it is tempting to lift your buttocks using the muscles at the back of your thighs, and your buttocks. Do not give in to this temptation! You should use your lower abs to lift your buttocks and use your upper abs to lift your shoulders.

Variation

At first, so you can learn to lift your buttocks using your lower abdominal muscles, simplify the exercise by keeping your shoulders on the floor. Once you have truly mastered the movement of the pelvis, then you can add your shoulders to the exercise.

NOTE

To feel this exercise more, keep your hands on your abs with your fingers on your lower abdomen.

RISKS

⚠ Be careful not to pinch discs in your lumbar and cervical spine. Raise yourself slowly, and do not make any jerky movements.

79

EXERCISES FOR THE UPPER ABDOMINAL MUSCLES
2 Sit-Up

This exercise works the abdominal wall and the hip flexors.

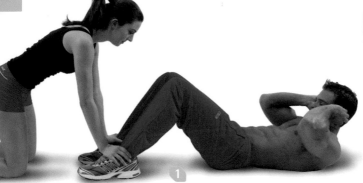

HELPFUL HINTS

The placement of your hands affects the difficulty of this exercise. Here are the positions in order from easiest to hardest (see also page 42):

- Arms straight out in front of your body
- Hands on your lower chest
- Hands on your shoulders
- Hands behind your head
- Straight arms behind your head

A good tapering set is to start sit-ups with your arms held out behind you. At failure, bring your hands behind your head, and so on. This way you can get a few more repetitions each time.

Lie on your back with your hands on your ears and your legs bent. Have a partner hold your feet, or you can tuck them under a machine or a bar ❶.

Slowly raise your shoulders to lift your torso off the floor. You should curl up just until your torso meets your thighs ❷. Hold this position and squeeze your abdominal muscles tightly. Return to your starting position and begin again, always without any abrupt movements.

A partner can pull you backward, especially during the descent ❸.

- Exhale during the contraction.
- Inhale as you lower your torso to the floor.

1. Performing the exercise

2. Variation with arms held straight out in front to make the exercise easier

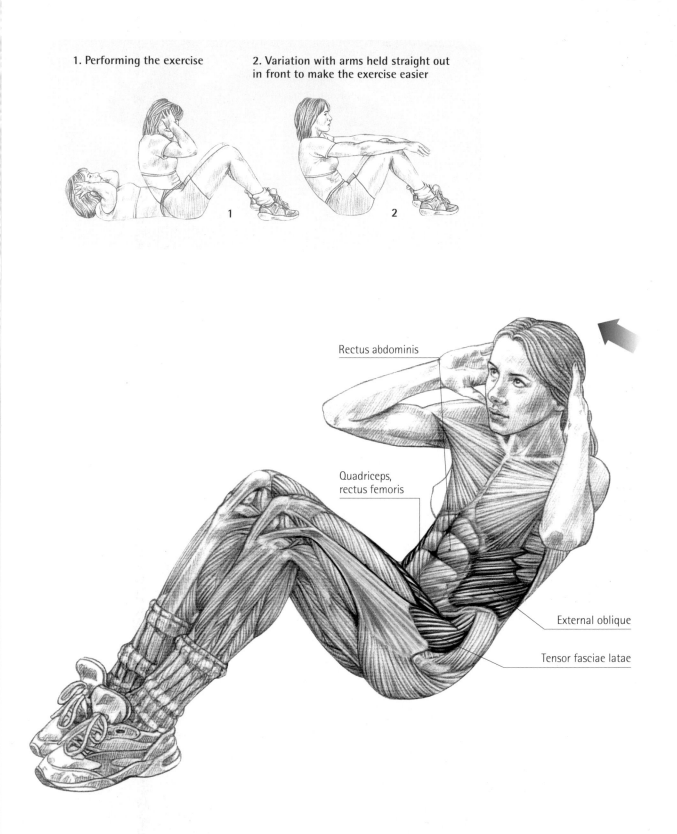

Rectus abdominis

Quadriceps, rectus femoris

External oblique

Tensor fasciae latae

d To have a little fun with this, you can combine sit-ups with throwing a medicine ball.

This exercise allows you to work on vigor in your muscles while increasing the resistance you must overcome to lift your torso. Throwing the ball is exceptionally good physical preparation if you play basketball or volleyball.

There are two main techniques for holding the ball in the lengthened position:

1. Beginning version: Hold the ball near the top of your chest.

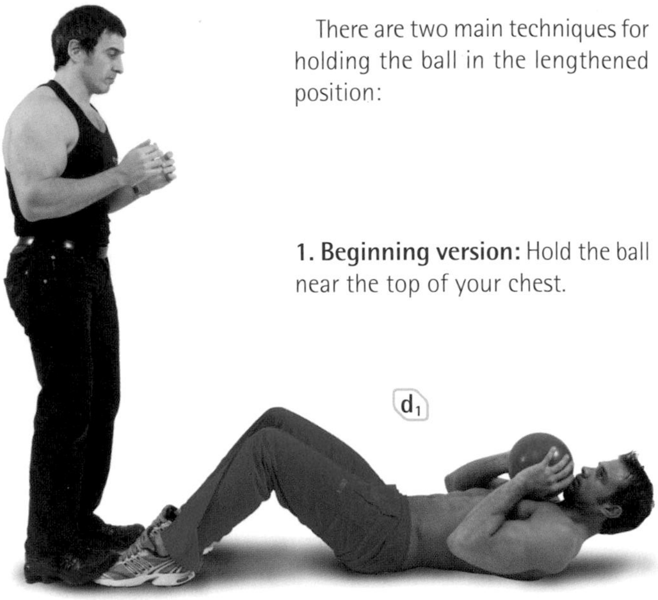

d₁

2. Advanced version: Hold the ball with your arms semistretched above your head.

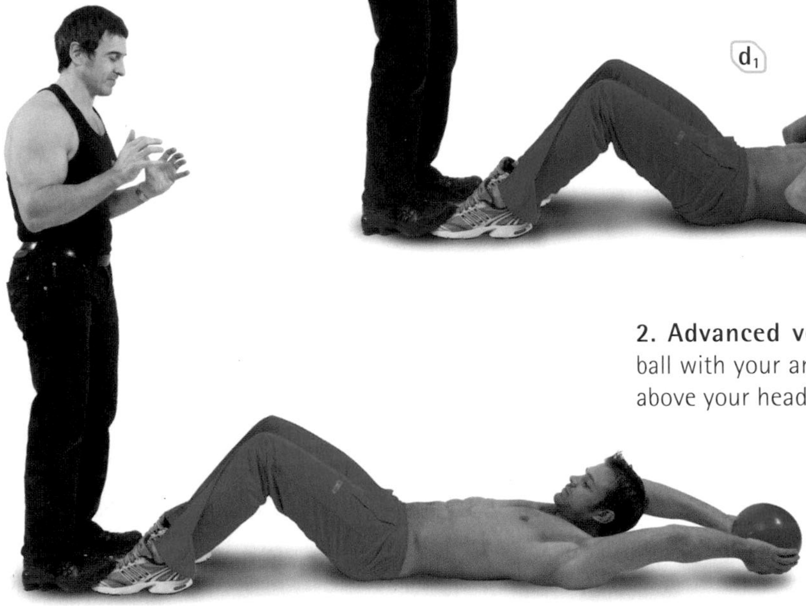

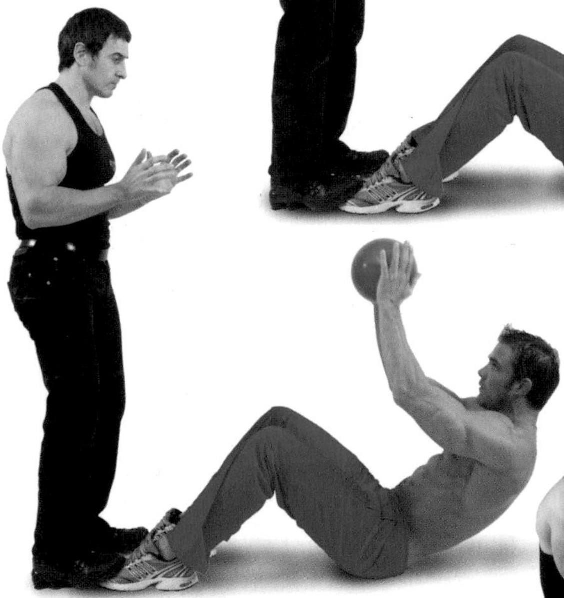

d₂

As you lift your torso, wind up your arms and throw the medicine ball as far as you possibly can. You must throw the ball before you reach the contracted position. Your partner stands on or near your feet as you sit up to catch the ball and returns it to you after you have lowered your torso.

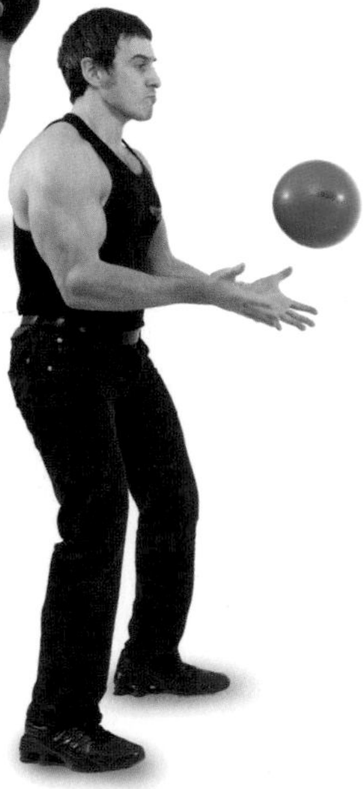

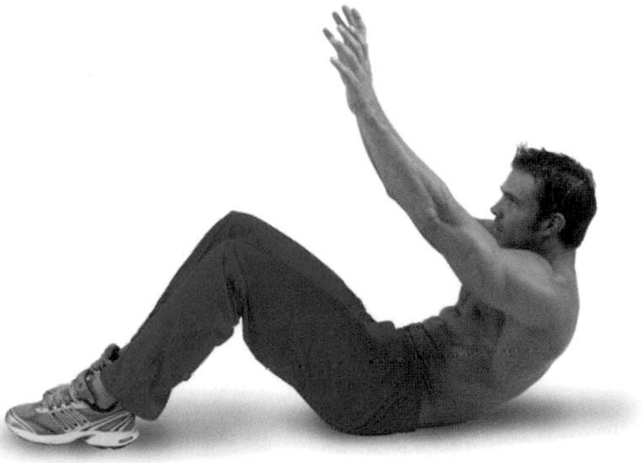

e⟩ Rather than bend the legs to 90 degrees, some people prefer to keep them straight. This accentuates the role of the hip flexors more.

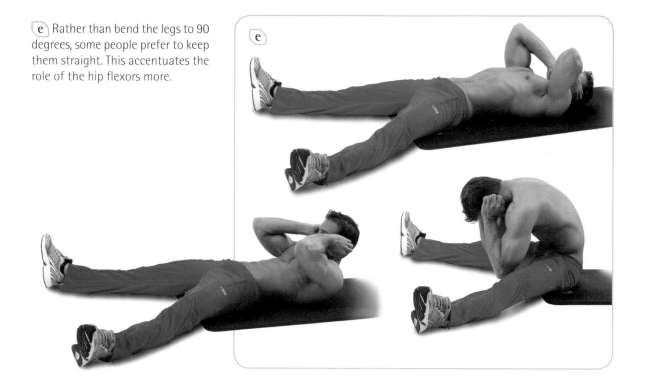

f⟩ Instead of coming up very straight, bring your right elbow toward your left knee to increase the work in the obliques. You can do either of the following:

- A rotation toward the left and then another toward the right for the next repetition
- All the rotations toward the left for a complete set before moving to a set with rotations to the right

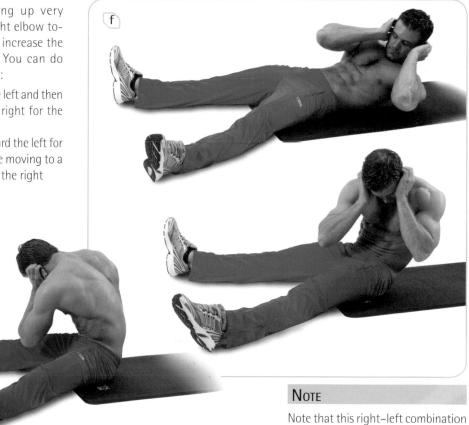

NOTE

Note that this right–left combination counts as only one set, not two sets.

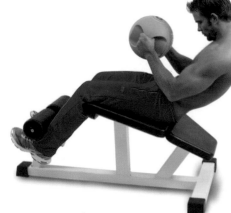

g You can also do this same rotation exercise on an ab bench using a weight.

ADVANTAGES

Sit-ups are especially good for runners who need powerful hip flexors to move quickly. For sports requiring running and torso rotation, you should do more sit-ups with rotation, as shown on this page.

DISADVANTAGES

The rectus abdominis is no longer the only muscle responsible for the movement, because the hip flexors steal the show. The more the legs help lift the torso, the less the abdominal muscles control the exercise.

RISKS

⚠ The lumbar spine is abused as the tension generated by the hip flexors increases. If you have even the slightest pain in your discs, you should not do this exercise.

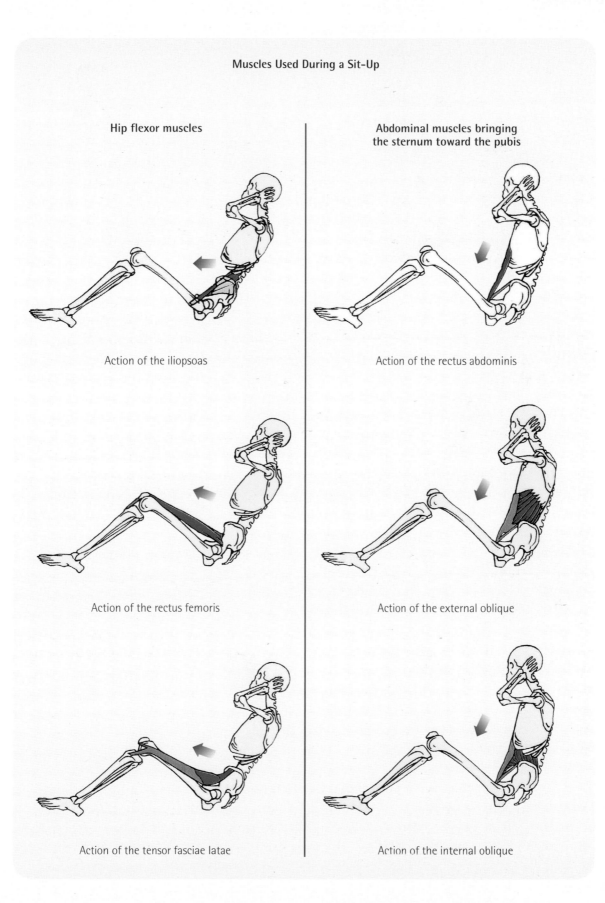

Hip flexor muscles

Abdominal muscles bringing
the sternum toward the pubis

Action of the iliopsoas

Action of the rectus abdominis

Action of the rectus femoris

Action of the external oblique

Action of the tensor fasciae latae

Action of the internal oblique

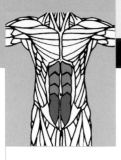

EXERCISES FOR THE LOWER ABDOMINAL MUSCLES

1 Pelvic Tilt on the Pull-Up Bar

This exercise helps you quickly learn how to contract your lower abdominal muscles.

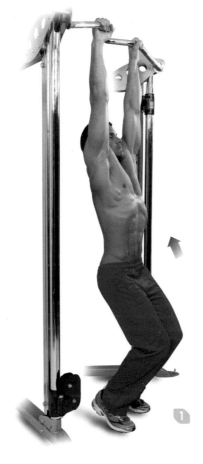

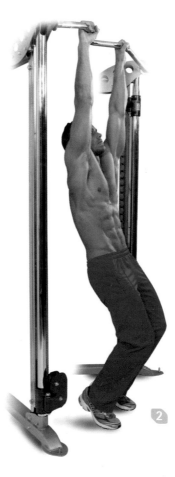

HELPFUL HINTS

Use only slight tension in your arms at first so that you can really become aware of the exercise as well as the work of your lower abdominal muscles. Arch your low back slightly while pulling back your buttocks. Come back to a straight position by moving your buttocks forward (tilting your pelvis backward), using only the strength of your lower abs. The mistake here would be to push on your legs to straighten your back.

With each additional set, put a little more weight onto your arms and also your abdominal muscles to make the exercise harder. However, be careful not to place too much resistance on your arms, because that could recruit other muscles that you are trying to relax. If that happens, your lower abdominal muscles will not learn to do this exercise correctly.

Hang from a pull-up bar with your hands shoulder-width apart in an overhand grip (thumbs facing each other). Your feet should be in front of your body with your toes on the floor. Your thighs form about a 120-degree angle with the floor ❶ and ❷. If the bar is too high, put your feet on a bench, chair, or stool.

Your feet should not support all of your body weight. You need a certain amount of tension in your arms, which you can regulate by pushing more or less on your legs.

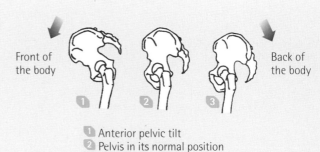

Front of the body

Back of the body

❶ Anterior pelvic tilt
❷ Pelvis in its normal position
❸ Posterior pelvic tilt

2 Leg Lift

This exercise helps you quickly learn how to contract your lower abdominal muscles.

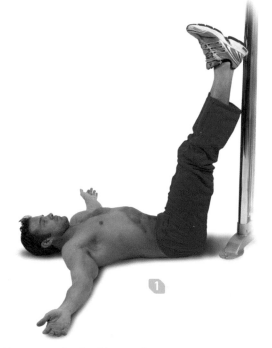 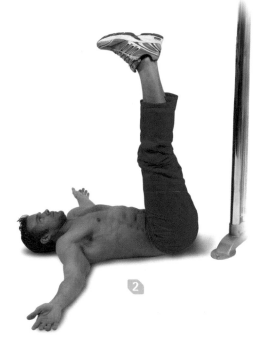

Lie on your back with your buttocks about 12 inches (30 cm) from a wall. Keep your legs straight and your heels against the wall ❶.

Using your lower abs, pull your thighs toward your head while lifting your buttocks until your legs are perpendicular to the floor ❷. Hold this contracted position for a few seconds before lowering your heels back to the wall.

The small range of motion in this exercise, as well as perfect control over the angles of movement, help recruit the lower abs. This prevents the hip flexors from intruding on the exercise.

More difficult version

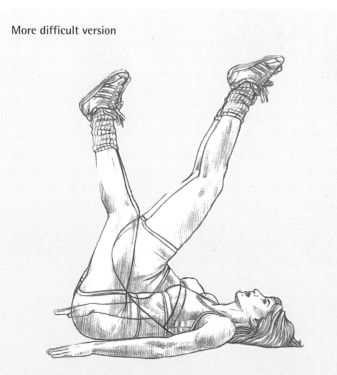

89

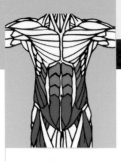

EXERCISES FOR THE LOWER ABDOMINAL MUSCLES
3 Hanging Leg Raise

This exercise works the entire abdominal wall but attempts to focus on the lower abdominal muscles in particular.

Of all the variations of leg raises (see pages 46 to 51), this one is the most difficult to do because of the great resistance the abdominal muscles are working against.

🖐 Hang from a pull-up bar with your hands about shoulder-width apart in an overhand grip (thumbs facing each other). Bring your legs to a 90-degree angle to your torso so that your thighs are parallel to the floor. This is your starting position **1** and **2**.

🖐 Use your lower abs to swing your pelvis forward and bring your knees toward your shoulders **3**. Lift your pelvis as high as possible by curling up as much as you can. Hold the contracted position for 1 second before lowering your pelvis. Be careful not to lower your legs below the parallel starting position.

HELPFUL HINTS

The hardest part of this exercise when you first try it is not swinging too much. In the other versions of leg raises described in part 4, your body is blocked by a hard surface (the floor or a bench). But when you are on a pull-up bar, there is nothing to stabilize you. With training, you will learn how to avoid swinging too much.

So that you do not lose your grip on the bar before your abs are done working, you can use ab straps to strengthen your grip on the pull-up bar (see page 94 on the lower left side).

⚠️ The most common mistake here is to start from a position where the knees are "looking" at the floor instead of a position where the thighs are parallel to the floor. Imagine a circle: The lower quarter of the circle works the hip flexors rather than the abdominal muscles. The abs work only in the upper quarter of the circle by lifting the thighs from a parallel position to a perpendicular position and bringing your knees as close as possible to your face.

Development

Before trying leg raises on a pull-up bar, it is best to first gain strength by working on the floor and then seated on a bench. If moving from the seated version to the pull-up bar version is too hard, you can use an incline ab bench to smooth the transition.

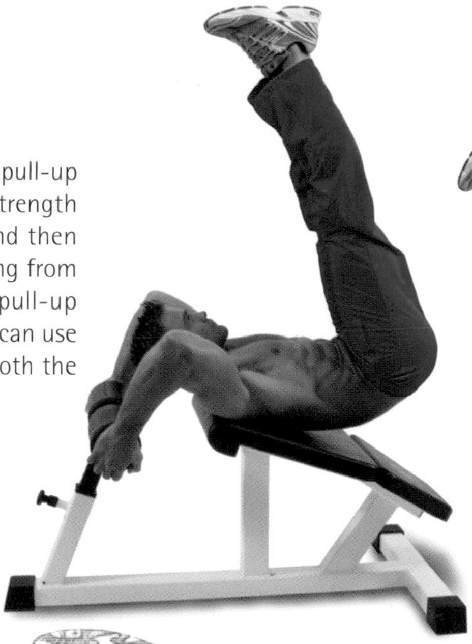

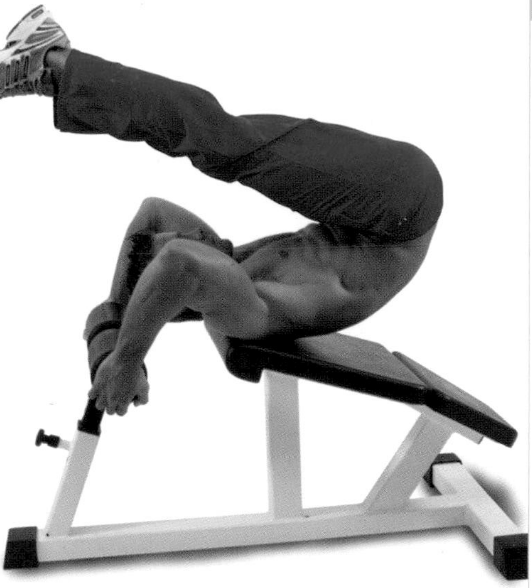

If you move from a small incline to a steep incline, your lower abs will get strong enough over time so that they can easily lift the weight of your legs on the pull-up bar.

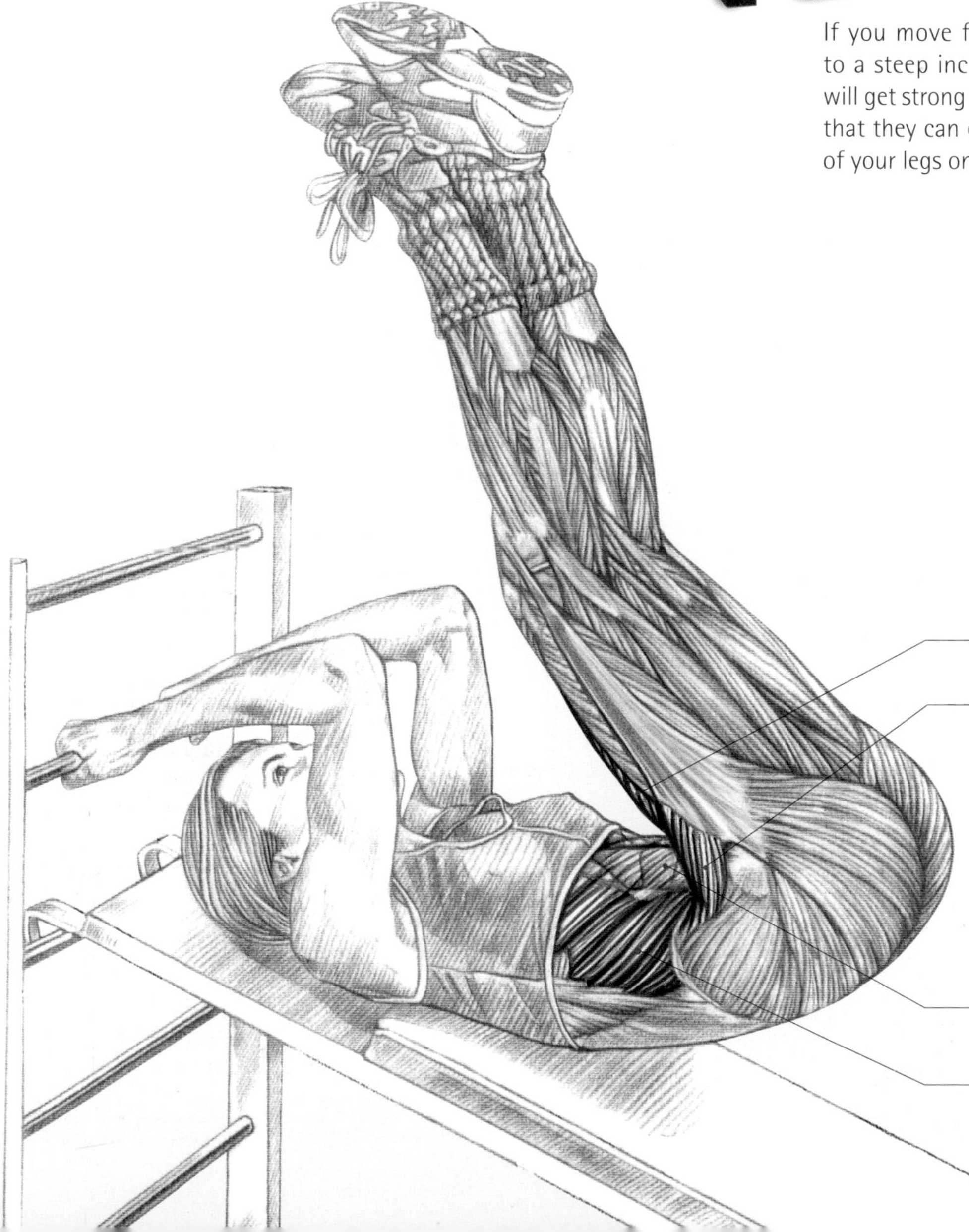

Quadriceps, rectus femoris

Tensor fasciae latae

Rectus abdominis

External oblique

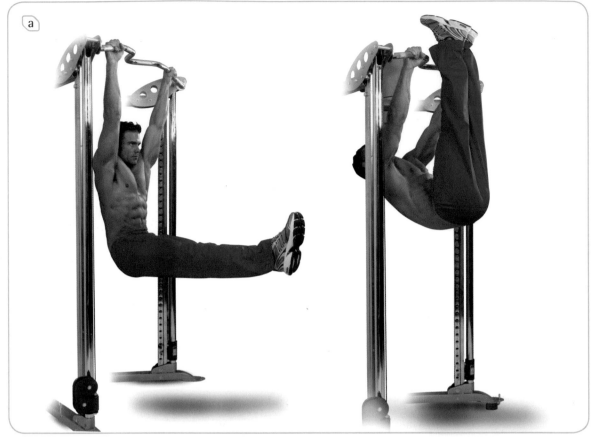

Variations

You can do any of the following:

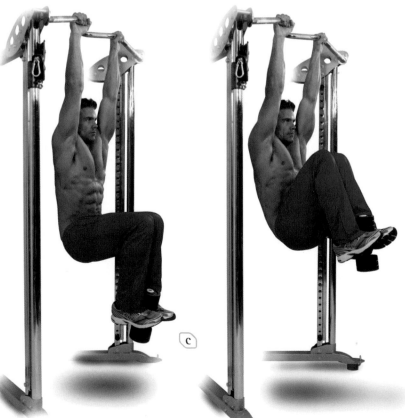

a Keep your legs straight (the exercise will be quite a bit harder).

b Bring your calves under your thighs (the exercise will be easier).
A good combination is to start the exercise with straight legs. When you reach fatigue, bend your legs so that you can get a few more repetitions.

c Hold a weight between your feet.

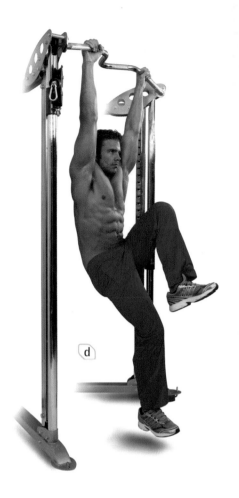

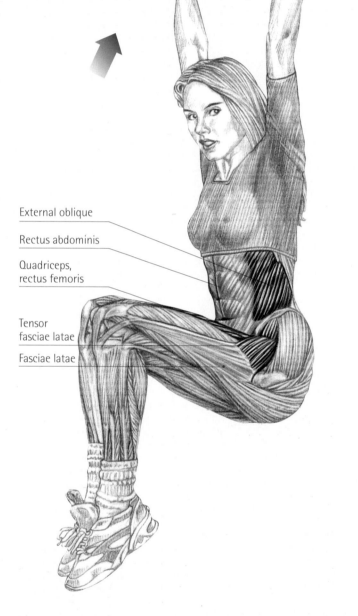

d To reduce the resistance your abs are working against, you can try to work only one leg at a time. But if you feel any pinching in your back, then this variation is not recommended.

External oblique

Rectus abdominis

Quadriceps, rectus femoris

Tensor fasciae latae

Fasciae latae

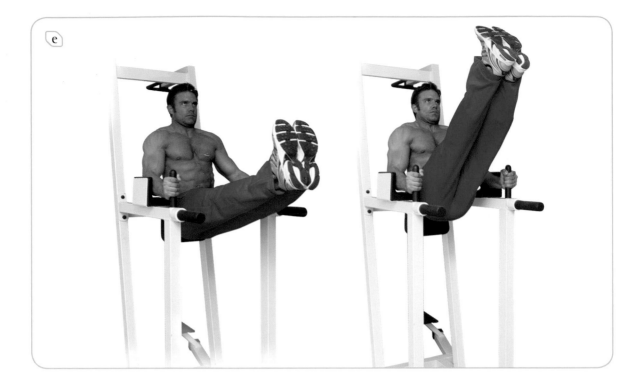

(e) You can use an ab chair to support yourself by your elbows instead of your hands. An ab chair is more stable and more comfortable than the pull-up bar.

(f) If one of these chairs is not available, you can use ab straps. You can use these to hang by your elbows and not your hands. This variation is also more comfortable than the pull-up bar. Since it is more difficult to swing from front to back, the exercise is more effective but also harder to do.

ADVANTAGES

The resistance placed on the lower abdominal muscles is at its maximum, which will help you progress quickly.

DISADVANTAGES

The major problem in isolating the lower abdominal muscles is the lack of strength in this part of the body. The fact that you have to lift your legs might prove to be too much resistance for you. As a result, you might tend to pull up however you can, but not with your lower abs. So it is easier to do this exercise incorrectly than it is to do it correctly. If you feel a pulling sensation in your low back, it means you are doing the exercise incorrectly. There is a certain learning curve required for this exercise.

RISKS

⚠ If your legs go lower than the parallel position, you will end up arching your low back. This is dangerous, and it also means that you are working the wrong muscles.

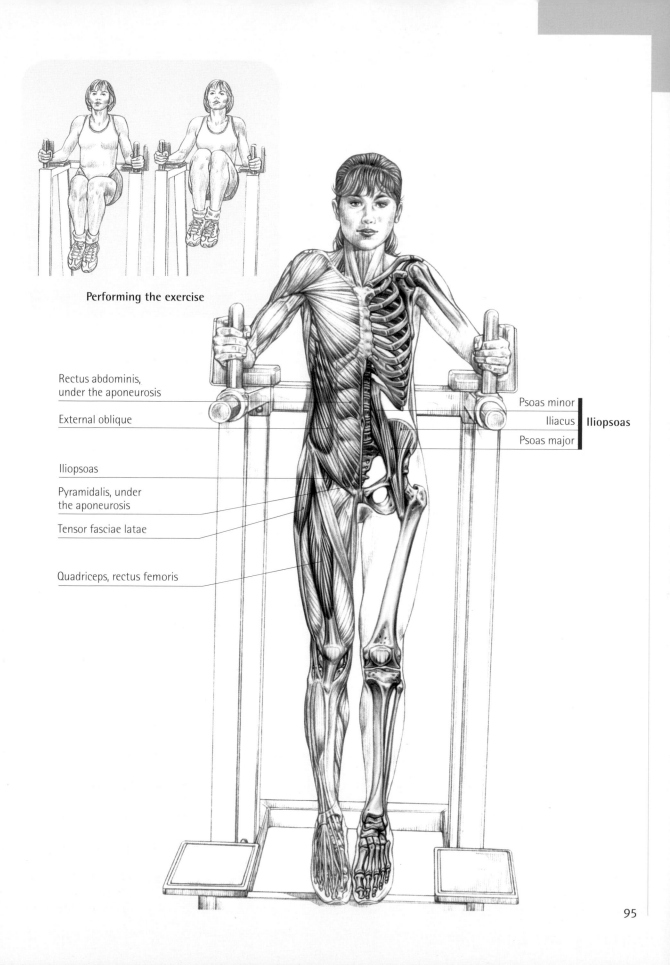

Performing the exercise

Rectus abdominis,
under the aponeurosis

External oblique

Iliopsoas

Pyramidalis, under
the aponeurosis

Tensor fasciae latae

Quadriceps, rectus femoris

Psoas minor
Iliacus   **Iliopsoas**
Psoas major

EXERCISES FOR THE OBLIQUES

1 Hanging Leg Raise to the Side

This exercise targets the obliques as well as the quadratus lumborum.

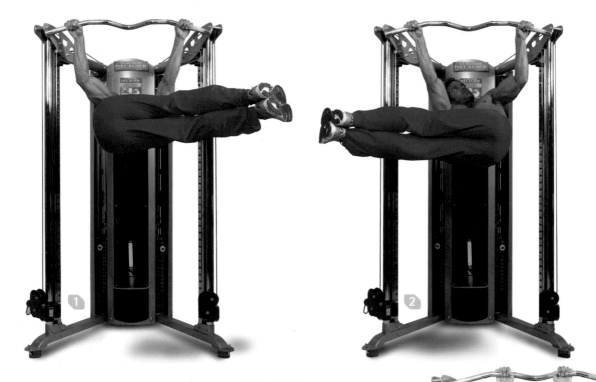

🔹 Hang from a pull-up bar with your hands about shoulder-width apart in an overhand grip (thumbs facing each other). Bring your legs to a 90-degree angle to your torso so that your thighs are parallel to the floor.

🔹 Using your obliques, swing your hips to the right. Lift them as high as you can while pushing your pelvis slightly forward. Hold the contracted position for 1 second before coming back down **1** and **2**.

Variations

a To decrease the resistance your obliques are working against, you can work only one leg at a time.

b You can keep your legs straight as shown above (the exercise will be quite a bit harder), or you can bring your calves under your thighs to make the exercise easier (see the top left corner of page 97).

c When the exercise gets too easy, you can hold a small weight between your feet.

Here is a good superset: Begin with hanging leg raises. When you reach failure, lie on the floor and continue the set with leg raises to the side.

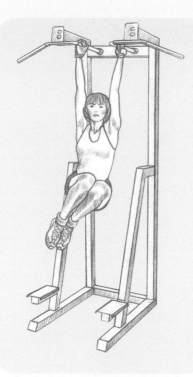

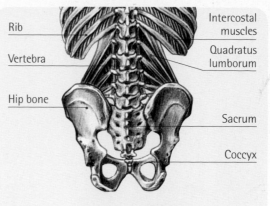

Quadratus lumborum

Quadratus lumborum

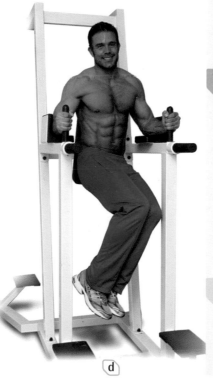

d

(d) The ab chair lets you hang by your elbows instead of your hands.

HELPFUL HINTS

Even though it is possible to do a repetition toward the right and then one to the left, you could end up using momentum and minimizing your muscle work. It is better to finish the set on the right before moving to the left side.

If you lack the strength, a high pulley (see page 108) can provide more appropriate resistance to help you gain the necessary strength to complete this exercise.

ADVANTAGES

Hanging leg raises are unrivaled in their ability to decompress the spine. Further, they are one of the rare exercises that strengthen the quadratus lumborum, a muscle that is indispensable in protecting the lumbar spine.

DISADVANTAGES

Some people will not be strong enough to do more than a few repetitions. In this case, a partner can support your legs to reduce the resistance on your obliques.

If you do not have a partner, you can bend just the working leg and keep the other in line with your body. You goal then will always be to support part of the weight of your thighs.

RISKS

⚠ To avoid injury to your discs, you should not swing your body or make any jerky movements as you raise your hips.

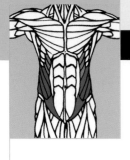

EXERCISES FOR THE OBLIQUES
2 Lying Twist

This exercise for the obliques attacks the love handles.

ADVANTAGES

Very few exercises target the muscles underneath the love handles.

DISADVANTAGES

If you have back problems, you should not do this exercise.

RISKS

⚠ Do not rotate too quickly or too far. Strive for a slow contraction over a short range of motion rather than an explosive movement over a wide range of motion.

Lie on your back with your arms out to your sides for stability, and bend your legs to 90 degrees **1**. Slowly lean your knees to the left only a few degrees at first **2**. Lower your legs farther with each repetition, only if you feel comfortable doing so.

Pause in the lengthened position before bringing your knees back up **3**. To maintain continuous tension, slowly return to the starting position and stop just before the knees are aligned with the torso. When you have finished a set for the right side, move to the left side.

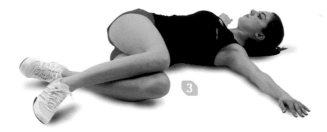

HELPFUL HINT

The right buttock will come off the floor when the knees lean to the left, but the left buttock remains in constant contact with the floor. Keep your head very straight on the floor and do not move your neck.

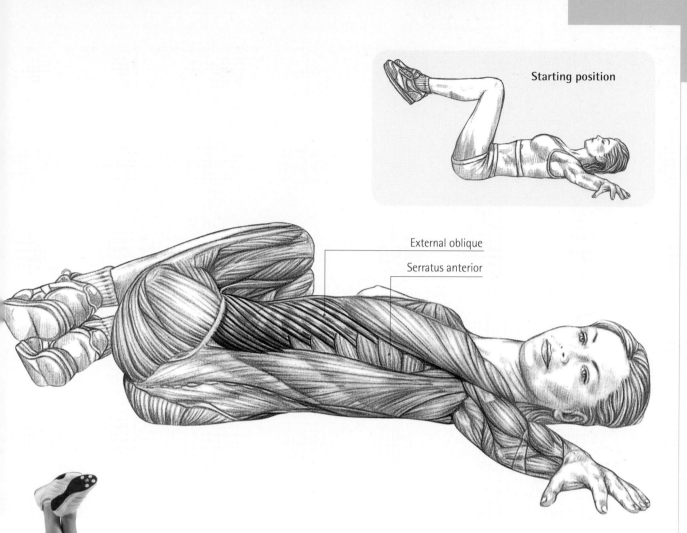

Starting position

External oblique

Serratus anterior

Note

You can also use these rotations as a stretch to relax the spine. In this case, there is no dynamic muscle work. Simply lower your left thigh to the floor and hold the stretch for 15 seconds to 1 minute. Then move to the right thigh.

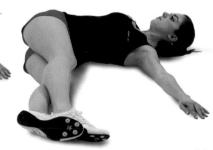

Variation

You can do these rotations with straight legs (this is the most difficult version).

PART 5

Exercises Using Machines and Accessories

The purpose of good ab machines is to provide the optimal trajectory for abdominal and core work. It is not always easy for a beginner to find the right trajectory for exercises that are done on the floor. In theory, machines should eliminate this learning period so that your workouts are immediately effective. Unfortunately, the abdominal muscles are among those that often fall victim to the abundance of poorly conceived machines. A poor ab machine will bend you in half by bringing your torso straight toward your thighs.

If the trajectory is poorly conceived, then the machine tries to make you do an exercise that is at best uncomfortable and at worst dangerous. On the contrary, a good machine helps you curl your spine, which brings your shoulders toward your lower abdomen and not toward your knees.

Purpose of Home Equipment

Many advertisements for core workouts and gadgets are on television today; they claim to give you rock-hard abs without any effort.

We need to debunk the myth that it is so easy to develop strong abdominal and core muscles. As users of these kinds of machines, we may want to believe this, but nothing is more untrue. The two main ingredients of a six-pack are an iron will and perseverance—in workouts as well as in your diet.

Fortunately, new tools are better, and better made. Some are still ineffective, even dangerous, but others are downright ingenious. This is why we mention here the best tools available, because they do have a place among the good exercises for the abdominal and core muscles.

The main interest in machines you can use at home is practicality. If you have a good machine, you no longer need to go to a gym to use a machine to help you work your abdominal and core muscles. Further, these machines are marketed as being fun to use.

The limiting factor of these gadgets is often their quality and the fact that you cannot make the exercise harder by adding additional weight once you get stronger. Even more, the fun aspect often fades after the first few uses, which explains why many of these tools end up in the back of the closet.

Professional Machines

The professional machines you find in the gym have three purposes:

1. Provide an optimal trajectory
2. Provide a wide variety of devices to alleviate the monotony of single exercises
3. Offer a wide array of resistances that are appropriate for beginners as well as advanced athletes

It is difficult to make the exercises you do on the floor more challenging by adding outside resistance. Even with a small weight, the center of gravity will shift, and this reduces the work of the abdominal muscles and increases the work of the hip flexors.

The main disadvantage of professional machines is that you must have a gym membership to use them. When you want to do only abdominal and core exercises, why pay for a full membership? And that does not include the time you lose in traveling to and from the gym. In this case, a home machine will have to suffice.

Even though machines have many advantages, this does not mean that

- you need them in order to do core work, or
- that using them will make it easy for you to get a six-pack.

Therefore, the core programs in part 6 consist almost exclusively of exercises that do not require any special equipment.

1 Machine Crunch

This exercise works the entire abdominal wall and especially the upper rectus abdominis.

There are three main types of crunch machines.

Type 1: You sit down to use this machine. Your torso leans forward, but your legs do not move. Adjust the weight as well as the height of the seat before you sit down. Put your feet flat on the floor or under the foot holds (if they are provided). The more the feet are held immobile, the more the hip flexors will come into play. However, you often need to anchor your legs if you do not want to fall out of the machine when using a heavy weight. Grab the handles of the machine and use your abdominal muscles (not your arms) to curl your torso forward. Stop as soon as you begin to bend your lumbar spine. Pause in this position while squeezing your abdominal muscles tightly. Slowly come back to the starting position but do not completely straighten your spine. Then begin the exercise again, always without making any jerky movements.

Type 2: You sit down to use this machine. Your torso leans forward, and your legs come toward your torso simultaneously. Your feet are not anchored; therefore, they are allowed to move. However, you are not able to move your feet so much that you could pull using your lower abs rather than your thighs, which involves the hip flexors. Other than this difference, the use of this machine is similar to the one just described.

Type 3: You lie down to use this machine, and your back is pressed into a bench. This machine is an advanced version of classic crunches. Using elbow supports, you move a pendulum, which holds weights so that you can adjust the difficulty of the exercise. Other than that, using this machine is similar to doing crunches.

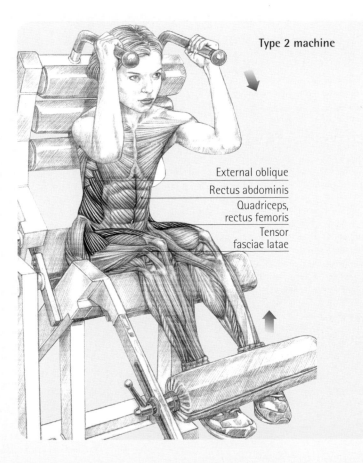

Type 2 machine

External oblique
Rectus abdominis
Quadriceps, rectus femoris
Tensor fasciae latae

ADVANTAGES

Heavy work is much easier if you use a machine. Athletes who need to strengthen both their abdominal muscles and their hip flexors will get the most benefit from these machines.

DISADVANTAGES

Among the classic models from the previous generation, you will find many more bad ab machines than good ab machines.

RISKS

⚠ Never let the machine arch your back. Forcibly arching your back repeatedly will damage your spine. Maintain continuous tension with your back slightly bent forward as you perform the exercise.

EXERCISES FOR THE UPPER ABDOMINAL MUSCLES

2 Swiss Ball Crunch

This exercise is an advanced version of classic crunches.
Lying on a Swiss ball has three benefits:

- More effective lumbar support than the floor since the ball mimics the curve of the vertebrae
- A better stretch for the abdominal muscles during the lower part of the movement
- A more intense contraction since the ball flattens as you come back up, which helps the back curve better

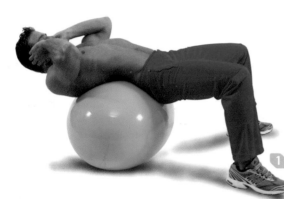 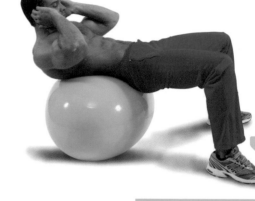

Lie with the middle of your back on the top of the ball. Bend your legs and spread them apart with your feet flat on the floor and your hands by your ears. Your buttocks and shoulders lean toward the back, but they always stay in contact with the Swiss ball **1**.

Lift your shoulders by curling your torso up **2**. Stop as soon as your lower lumbar spine starts to come off the ball. Pause in this position while tightly squeezing your abdominal muscles. Slowly return to the starting position and then begin again, always without any jerky movements.

HELPFUL HINT

It is better for the Swiss ball to rest on a base so that it does not move when you lift your torso. If you do not have a base, you can ask a partner to hold the ball so that it does not get away.

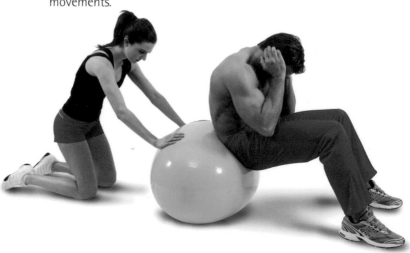

a You can also use a Bosu ball. It has the same benefits as a Swiss ball, but it is more stable. It might not allow you to work on your balance, but it will help you avoid falling.

b The Swiss ball is highly appropriate for working on side rotation. Using it will allow you to straighten your torso better, which improves your ability to rotate your torso.

This gives you a more complete contraction than you could get from a floor exercise.

However, this is the version where the ball is most likely to slip if it is not well anchored to the floor.

ADVANTAGES

The range of motion in this exercise is more than double that of classic crunches, which makes abdominal work more effective.

RISKS

⚠ Do not overdo the stretch provided by this exercise. If the ball is not securely anchored to the floor, you might end up doing a somersault.

c To get an extremely wide range of motion, do sit-ups on the ball instead of crunches.

d If you do not have a Swiss ball, lie down across a weight bench. The majority of your torso and your buttocks hang off the bench. The increase in your range of motion is potentially greater than with a ball, but the position is less comfortable and your back is not supported as well.

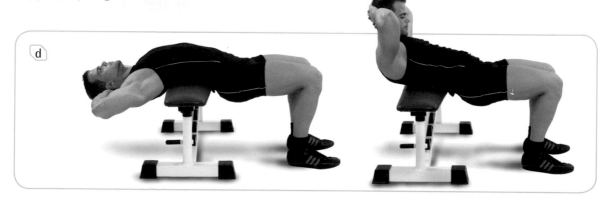

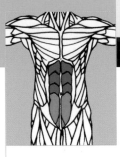

EXERCISES FOR THE UPPER ABDOMINAL MUSCLES
3 Rocking Machine Crunch

This exercise works the entire abdominal wall and especially the upper rectus abdominis.

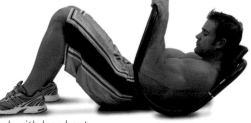

🖐 Lie on your back with legs bent, feet flat on the floor, and hands on the upper part of the machine. Press your neck firmly into the head rest.

🖐 Slowly curl your torso to lift your shoulders off the floor, and let the machine guide your trajectory. You need to come up as high as possible while keeping your lumbar spine pressed into the floor. Pause in the upper position and tightly squeeze your abdominal muscles. Slowly return to the starting position and then begin again, always without making any abrupt movements.

- Exhale during the contraction.
- Inhale as you lower your torso to the floor.

Variations

a) A partner can push on the handles to increase the resistance your muscles have to overcome.

HELPFUL HINT

The goal is to raise your torso using your abdominal muscles and not your arms. So your hands should not push on the handles. They are just barely holding on so that they cannot interfere, except at the end of the exercise if you need to use them to get a few more repetitions.

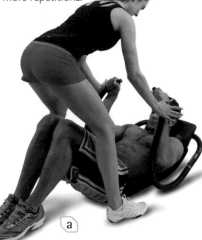

a

ADVANTAGES

You will feel your abdominal muscles working right away.

DISADVANTAGES

You must have one of these machines in order to use it. And it is a good bet that some people who own these machines never use them.

RISKS

⚠ If you are not using your hands or momentum to go too high, then this machine can help you work very safely. But if you push with your hands and your torso does not follow, then your neck may suffer from whiplash.

b) If you lie on your side, this exercise will better target your obliques.

c) To make this exercise harder, put a small metal weight plate between your head and the machine. Put a folded towel between you and the weight to make it more comfortable. Be careful that the weight does not slip and hit your neck during the exercise.

b

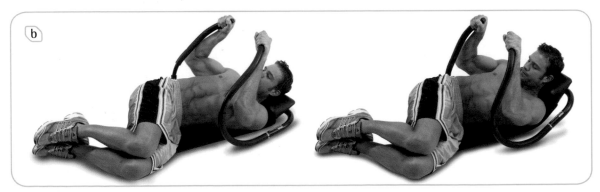

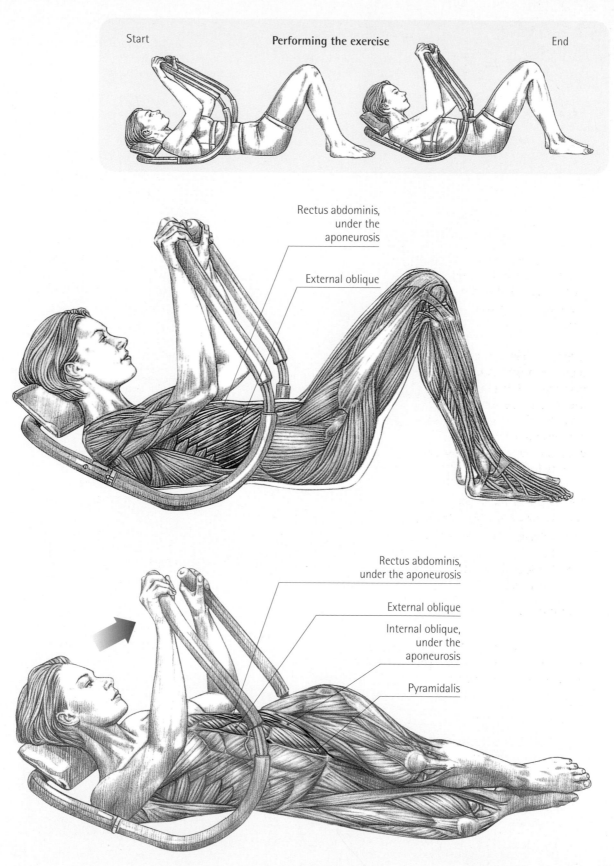

Rectus abdominis,
under the
aponeurosis

External oblique

Rectus abdominis,
under the aponeurosis

External oblique

Internal oblique,
under the
aponeurosis

Pyramidalis

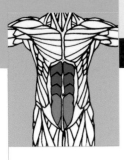

EXERCISES FOR THE UPPER ABDOMINAL MUSCLES
4 Standing Cable Crunch

This exercise works the entire abdominal wall and especially the upper rectus abdominis.

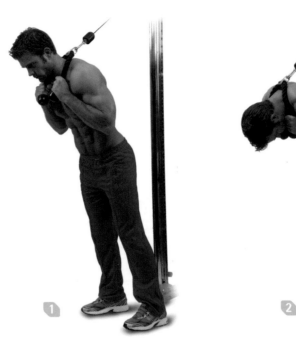

Stand with a high pulley behind you. Grab the cable rope attachment with your fingers facing your torso ❶.

Variation

Get on your knees with a high pulley behind you. Grab the bar attachment with your thumbs facing each other (see illustration on the next page). In both cases, slowly curl your chest in order to lean your torso slightly forward.

Bend down about 8 to 12 inches (20-30 cm) ❷. Pause in the contracted position. Slowly return to the starting position, but always keep your back slightly bent. Then begin again without making any jerky movements.

HELPFUL HINT

Avoid twisting your shoulders from right to left when you have trouble doing an additional repetition at the end of a set.

ADVANTAGES

The pulley helps you adjust the resistance in the exercise perfectly.

DISADVANTAGES

Beyond a certain weight, it becomes difficult to stay in place and precisely control the trajectory of your torso as you come back up.

RISKS

⚠ If the weight is controlling the exercise, you could move about randomly in the best case, and in the worst case you could injure yourself.

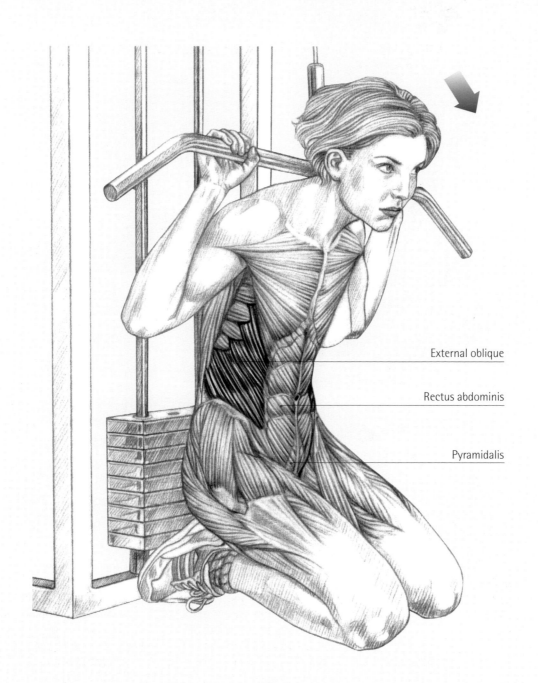

External oblique

Rectus abdominis

Pyramidalis

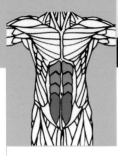

EXERCISES FOR THE LOWER ABDOMINAL MUSCLES
1 Ab Coaster

This machine works the entire abdominal wall and especially the lower abdominal muscles.

🟤 Get on your knees on the seat of the machine with your forearms anchored in the elbow holders and your hands gripping the handles 🟤. Move the seat along the rails using your lower abdominal muscles and not your thighs. Come up as high as possible while tucking in your abdomen 🟤.

🟤 Try to bring your lower abs up to your chest. The goal is not for them to touch, but as you concentrate on this imaginary goal it will help you achieve the proper trajectory of the exercise. Pause in the uppermost position while tightly squeezing your lower abdominal muscles. Lower yourself back to the starting position slowly and stop before your feet are perpendicular to the floor so that you can maintain continuous tension.

Variations

a If the exercise seems too difficult, you can put a foot on the floor to decrease the resistance.

HELPFUL HINTS

Even though the goal of the Ab Coaster is to provide the right trajectory to target your lower abs, there is no guarantee. You only have to look at the many advertisements to be convinced. The models willingly perform the exercise using their legs and not their abs. We do not advise you to copy the models.

The most common mistake is to put the entire weight of your body on the seat, which will require the hip flexors to intervene and compensate for the lack of strength in the lower abs. But if you really grip the handles, you will lighten the load on your abdominals. This is better at first so that you can learn to do the exercise correctly.

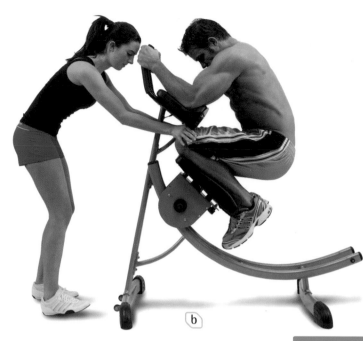

b

b To increase the difficulty of the exercise once you are stronger, you have some options:

- Add small weights underneath the seat.
- A partner can also push on your knees as the seat is returning to the starting position.

c By turning the seat to the side, you can target your obliques as well as your abdominal muscles.

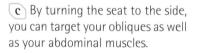

c

NOTE

Do not look up in the air. To roll up perfectly, keep your head leaning forward and do not move your neck.

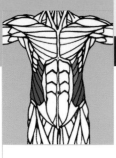

EXERCISES FOR THE OBLIQUES

1 Cable Twist
(Machine or Resistance Band)

This exercise targets the obliques, which helps with love handles. You must do this exercise unilaterally to create significant resistance for the muscle.

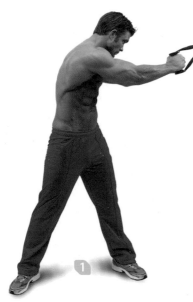

🖐 Adjust the pulley to midheight. Stand with the machine on your left and grab the left handle with your hands. Step to the side and away from the machine **1**.

🖐 Keep your legs apart for more stability and begin twisting from left to right. Do not twist your torso more than 45 degrees **2** and **3**. When you have finished the right side, you can move on to the left side.

HELPFUL HINTS

Without resistance from the side, twists have no purpose. Frenetically twisting with a bar on your shoulders serves no purpose, except to wear down your spine. The stress on your lumbar discs is even worse if you have a weighted bar on your shoulders.

The higher you place the pulley, the more you work your internal oblique. The lower you place the pulley, the more you work the external oblique.

Variations

a If you do not have an adjustable pulley, you can kneel in order to use the lower handle of the machine.

b Some machines are made for twisting (see the next page). If you use one, be sure that when you start twisting you do it gently. If you start roughly and initiate the movement with a jerk, you could move a vertebra.

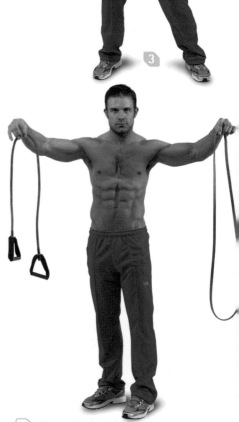

c If you do not have access to a cable machine, you can do these twists with a resistance band. Just attach it to a fixed point at midheight.

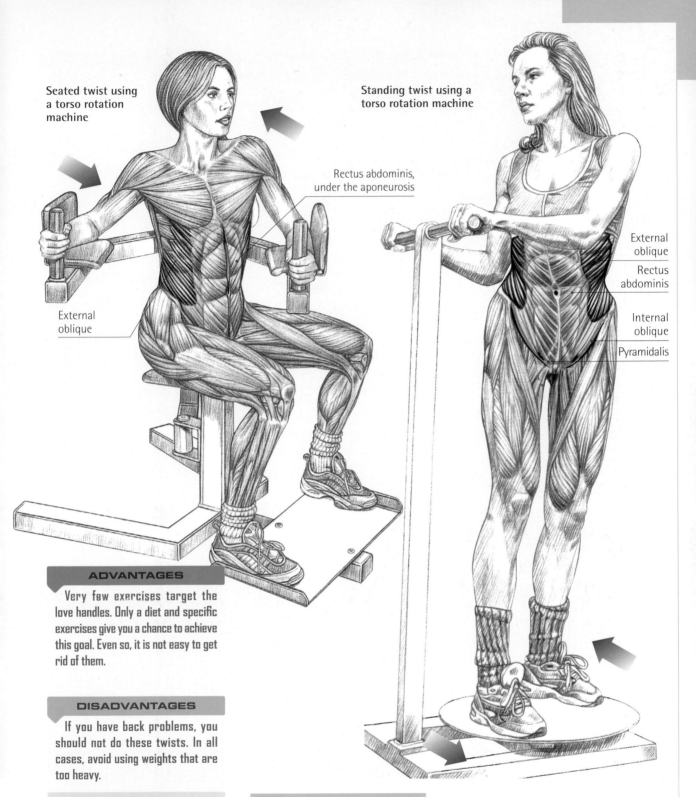

Seated twist using a torso rotation machine

Standing twist using a torso rotation machine

Rectus abdominis, under the aponeurosis

External oblique

External oblique

Rectus abdominis

Internal oblique

Pyramidalis

ADVANTAGES

Very few exercises target the love handles. Only a diet and specific exercises give you a chance to achieve this goal. Even so, it is not easy to get rid of them.

DISADVANTAGES

If you have back problems, you should not do these twists. In all cases, avoid using weights that are too heavy.

RISKS

⚠ Do not exaggerate the twists or do them too quickly. Strive for a very slow contraction over a short range of motion rather than an explosive movement over a large range of motion.

NOTES

This is an exercise that should be done slowly in long sets (25 repetitions). To get rid of love handles, you can do two to four sets (with no rest breaks) every day.

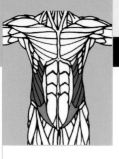

EXERCISES FOR THE OBLIQUES
2 Side Bend

This is an exercise that targets the obliques.
You must do this exercise unilaterally to create significant resistance for the muscle.

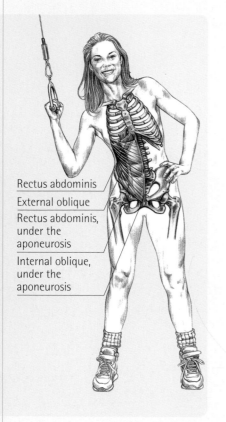

Rectus abdominis

External oblique

Rectus abdominis, under the aponeurosis

Internal oblique, under the aponeurosis

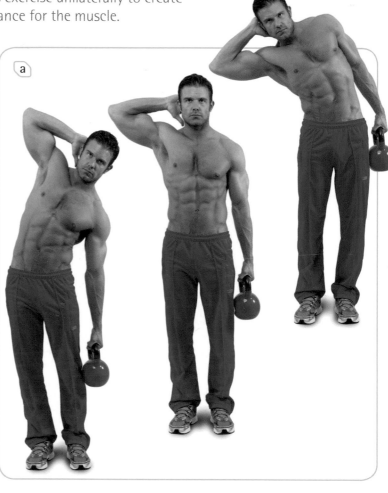

a

Attach a handle to a high pulley. Stand with the machine on your right and grab the handle with your right hand. Put your left hand on your hip to help your balance. Take a small step to the side away from the machine and keep your legs apart (see illustration above).

Bend to the side without going farther than 45 degrees. Stay in the low position while tightly squeezing your obliques before you straighten your torso. When you have finished the right side, you can move to the left side.

Variations

a Using a dumbbell: Instead of using a low pulley, the resistance is provided by a dumbbell or kettlebell. This variation has the same disadvantage as the next one in that it can put pressure on your back. Be careful when doing side bends with a dumbbell. These exercises are useful only in strength sports where a large amount of pressure is placed on the spine.

The most counterproductive way to work the obliques is to hold a dumbbell in each hand and swing from right to left. This swinging is caused by a pendulum effect. It does not use the strength of your obliques, it compromises the spine unnecessarily, and it still does not work your muscles.

b Using a low pulley: This exercise is easier to perform with a low pulley, but it still compromises the spine unnecessarily. However, doing this same exercise with a high pulley will actually relax the spine.

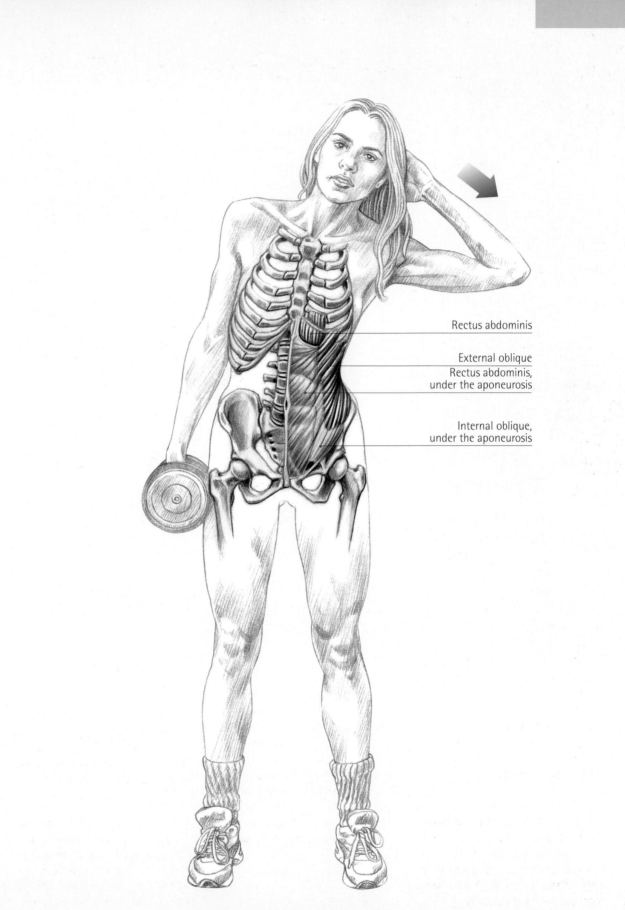

Rectus abdominis

External oblique
Rectus abdominis,
under the aponeurosis

Internal oblique,
under the aponeurosis

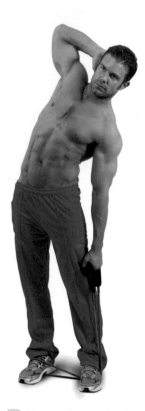
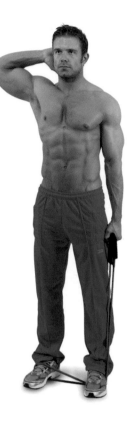
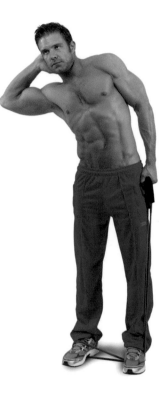

c Use a resistance band to get better continuous tension.

ADVANTAGES

Getting powerful obliques is necessary in strength sports or in twisting sports. In this case, side bends are a very helpful exercise.

DISADVANTAGES

For most people, side bends are redundant because of other exercises, like side crunches.

RISKS

⚠ You should not do too many side bends since they can be rough on your intervertebral discs. Do not bend abruptly or in an exaggerated manner. Rather, strive for a slow contraction over a small range of motion.

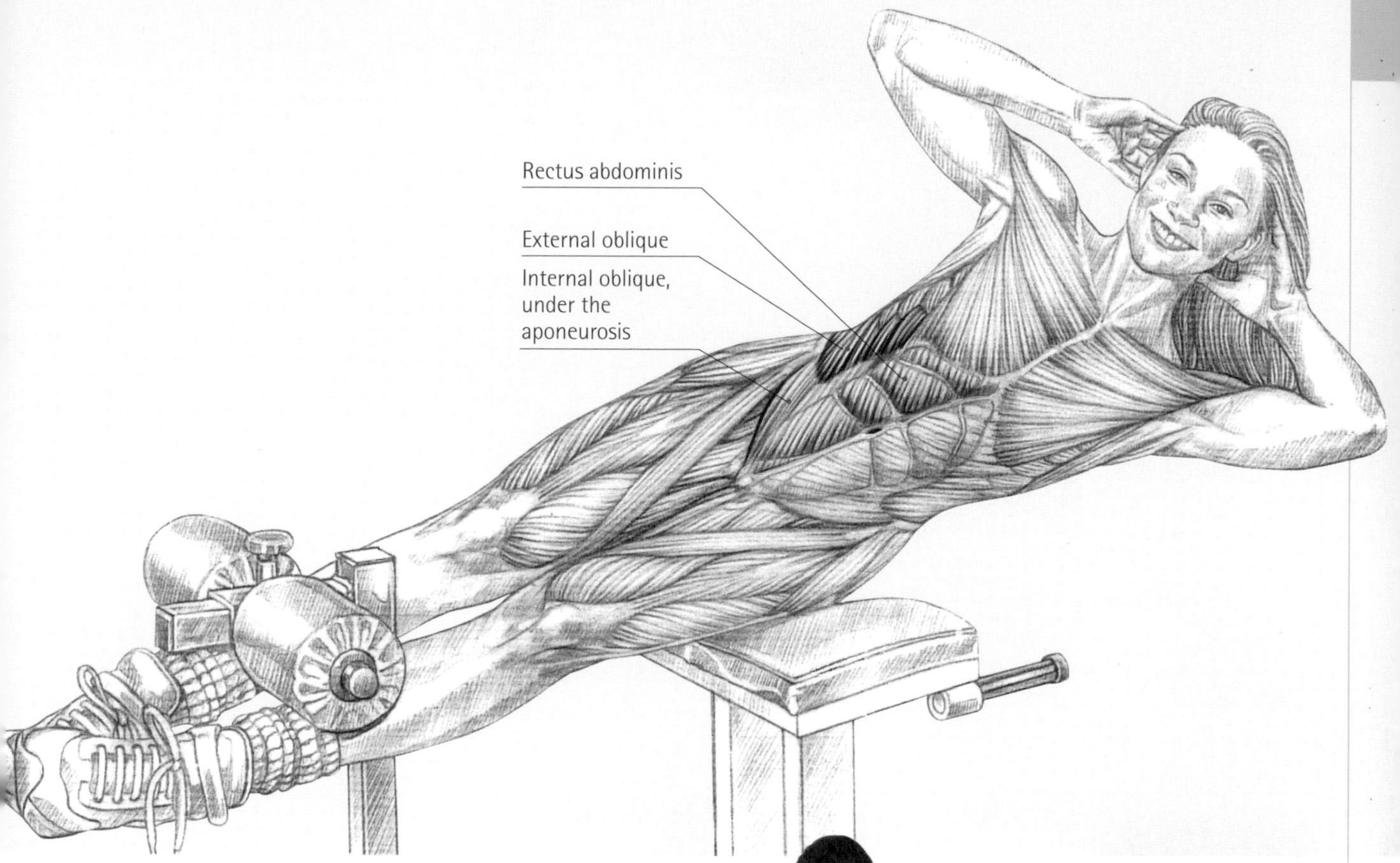

Rectus abdominis

External oblique

Internal oblique,
under the
aponeurosis

d Using a flat bench or a back bench: This is a very advanced exercise. Lie on your side on a bench with your feet anchored by the machine or by a partner and your upper body off the bench. Lean to the side a few degrees before raising yourself as high as you can. With each repetition, lower an inch more, but do not bend your torso beyond a 45-degree angle.

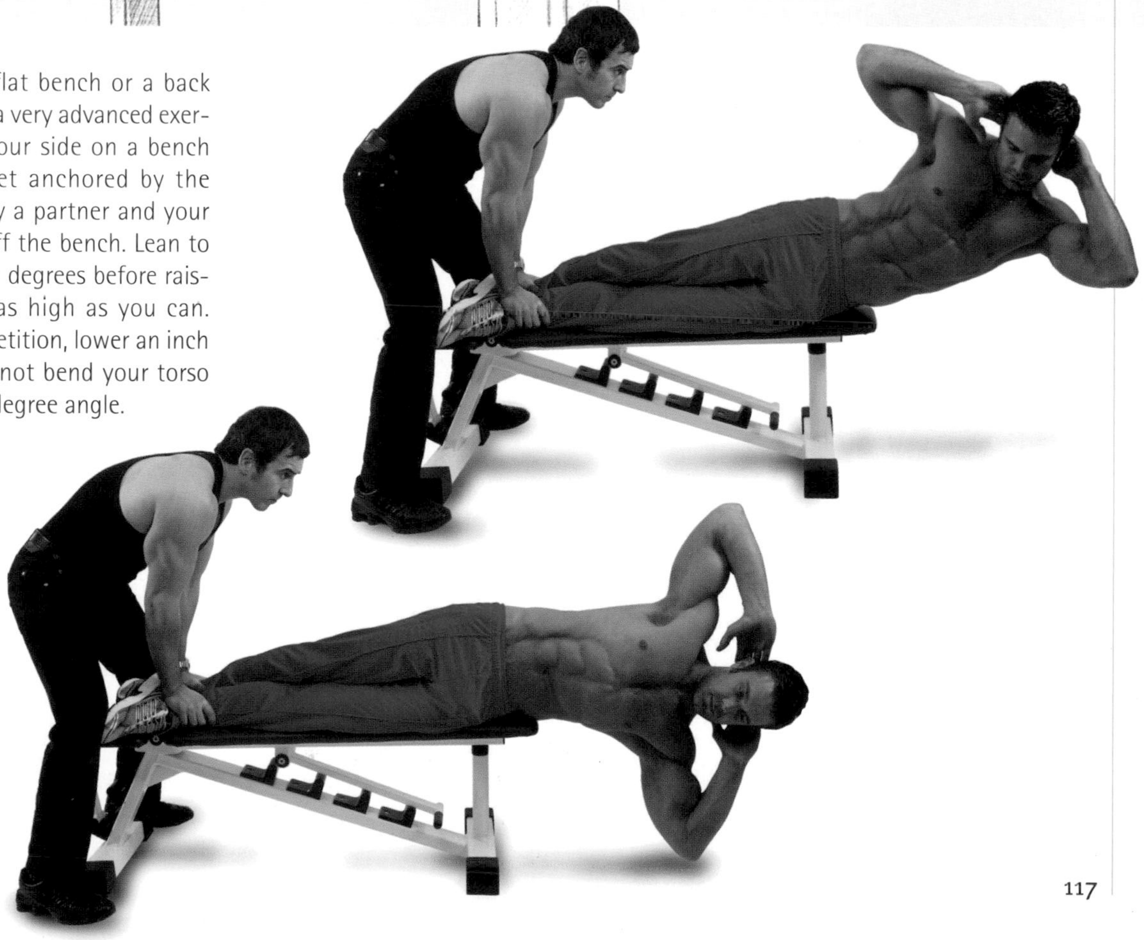

PART 6

Workout Programs

for Abdominal and Core Muscles

SIX-PACK PROGRAMS

HOW TO INTEGRATE ABDOMINAL AND CORE WORK INTO A TOTAL-BODY WORKOUT

There are five ways to integrate abdominal and core work into a general conditioning workout:

1. Begin your workouts with abdominal and core exercises as a warm-up.
2. End some of your workouts with abdominal and core work in conjunction with back decompression exercises.
3. Begin and end your workouts with abdominal and core exercises so that you increase the volume of work for your abs and core.
4. Do abdominal and core work in the morning and the evening, or even in the morning and evening at your home, since this work does not require a lot of equipment.
5. Do abdominal and core circuits in the morning and evening as well as before and after your workouts for other muscle groups. This will help you lose fat quickly.

Options 1 and 2 are perfect if you are a beginner. As you progress, you can increase the number of workouts that include abdominal and core exercises. So if you are an intermediate-level athlete, you can choose option 3. If you are an advanced athlete, you can integrate abdominal and core exercises before and after workouts and even do a little bit more at home.

Beginning Programs

One Workout per Week

● Crunch   p. 40
   5 sets of 20 to 15 repetitions with 30 seconds of rest between sets.

Two Workouts per Week

● Crunch   p. 40
   4 sets of 20 to 15 repetitions with 30 seconds of rest between sets.

● Lying leg raise   p. 46
   2 sets of 12 to 8 repetitions with 45 seconds of rest between sets.

Three Workouts per Week

● Crunch   p. 40
   3 sets of 20 to 15 repetitions with 30 seconds of rest between sets.

● Lying leg raise   p. 46
   3 sets of 12 to 8 repetitions with 45 seconds of rest between sets.

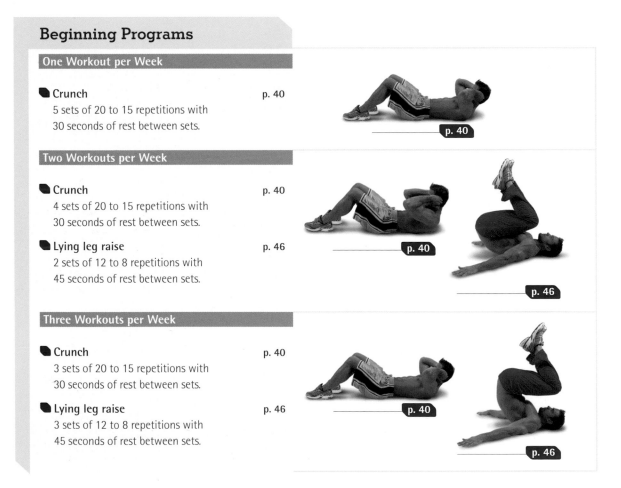

p. 40

p. 40

p. 46

p. 40

p. 46

Advanced Programs

Three Workouts per Week

Hanging leg raise   p. 90
4 sets of 12 to 8 repetitions with
45 seconds of rest between sets.

Crunch   p. 40
3 sets of 15 to 10 repetitions with
30 seconds of rest between sets.

Side crunch   p. 56
2 sets of 30 to 20 repetitions with
no rest between the right and left sides.

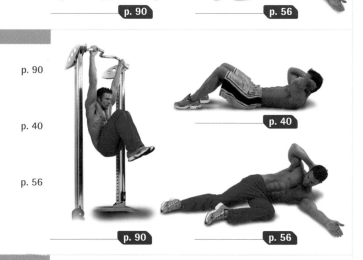

p. 40

p. 90

p. 56

Four Workouts per Week

Hanging leg raise   p. 90
3 sets of 12 to 8 repetitions with
45 seconds of rest between sets.

Crunch   p. 40
3 sets of 15 to 10 repetitions with
30 seconds of rest between sets.

Side crunch   p. 56
2 sets of 30 to 20 repetitions with
no rest between the right and left sides.

p. 40

p. 90

p. 56

Five Workouts per Week

Hanging leg raise   p. 90
3 sets of 12 to 8 repetitions with
45 seconds of rest between sets.

Double crunch   p. 79
3 sets of 12 to 8 repetitions with
30 seconds of rest between sets.

Side crunch   p. 56
2 sets of 30 to 20 repetitions with
no rest between the right and left sides.

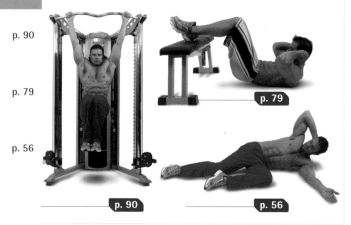

p. 79

p. 90

p. 56

SIX-PACK PROGRAMS

Very Advanced Programs

Three Workouts per Week

🔹 **Hanging leg raise**   p. 90
Do 15 to 8 repetitions;
at fatigue, combine with

🔹 **Lying leg raise**   p. 46
Do the maximum number of repetitions:
5 sets with 1 minute of rest between sets.

🔹 **Double crunch with weight on the torso**   p. 44
12 to 8 repetitions; at fatigue, put down the
weight so you can immediately combine with

🔹 **Classic crunch**   p. 40
Do the maximum number of repetitions:
5 sets with 45 seconds of rest between sets.

🔹 **Side crunch**   p. 56
5 sets of 20 to 15 repetitions with
no rest between the right and left sides.

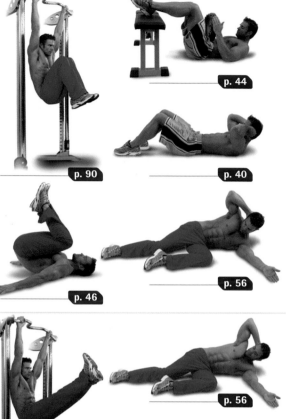

p. 44

p. 90

p. 40

p. 46

p. 56

Four Workouts per Week
WORKOUT 1

🔹 **Hanging leg raise with straight legs**   p. 92
15 to 10 repetitions; at fatigue,
bend your legs. Then, combine
immediately with

🔹 **Lying leg raise**   p. 46
Do the maximum number of repetitions:
6 sets with 1 minute of rest between sets.

🔹 **Side crunch**   p. 56
5 sets of 20 to 15 repetitions with
no rest between the right and left sides.

🔹 **Cable twist**   p. 112
A set to the right and then a set to the left
with no rest between the two:
5 sets of 20 to 15 repetitions.

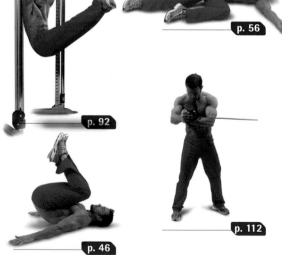

p. 56

p. 92

p. 112

p. 46

WORKOUT 2

🔹 **Double crunch with weight on the torso**   p. 44
25 to 8 repetitions; at fatigue, put down the
weight so you can immediately combine with

🔹 **Classic crunch**   p. 40
Do the maximum number of repetitions:
6 sets with 45 seconds of rest between sets.

p. 44

p. 40

● Twisting crunch — p. 54

5 sets of 20 to 15 repetitions with
no rest between the right and left sides.

● Cable twist — p. 112

A set to the right and then a set to the left
with no rest between the two:
5 sets of 20 to 15 repetitions.

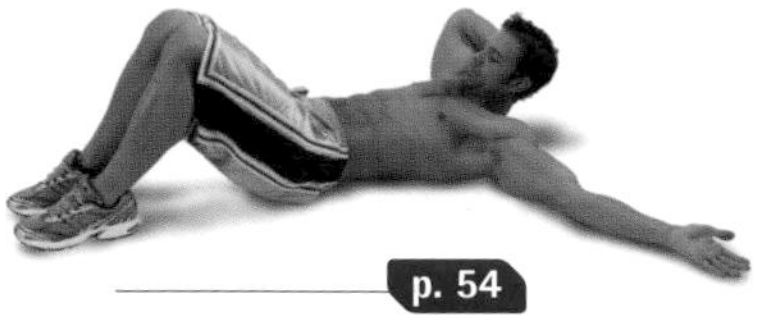

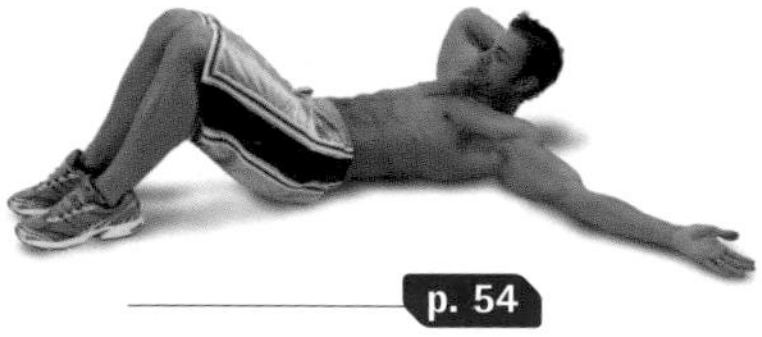

p. 54

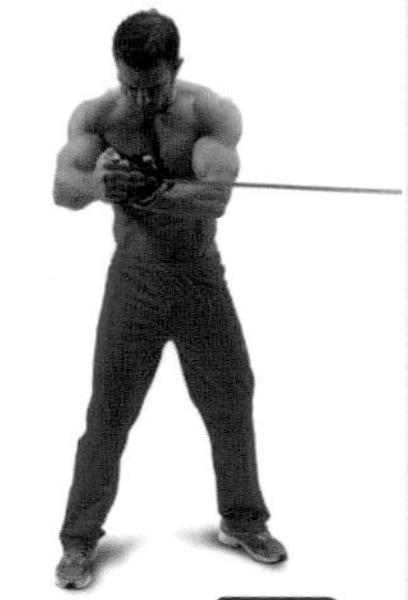

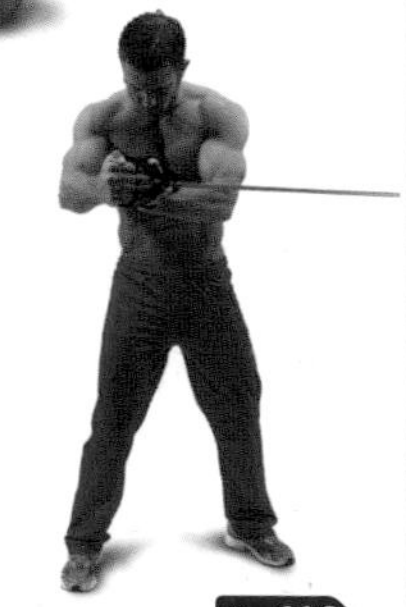

p. 112

WORKOUT 3: Repeat the cycle.

Five Workouts per Week

WORKOUT 1

● **Hanging leg raise with straight legs** — p. 92

15 to 10 repetitions; at fatigue,
bend your legs. Then, combine
immediately with

● **Lying leg raise** — p. 46

Do the maximum number of repetitions:
5 sets with 1 minute of rest between sets.

● **Side crunch** — p. 56

4 sets of 20 to 15 repetitions with
no rest between the right and left sides.

● **Cable twist** — p. 112

A set to the right and then a set to the left
with no rest between the two:
4 sets of 50 to 30 repetitions.

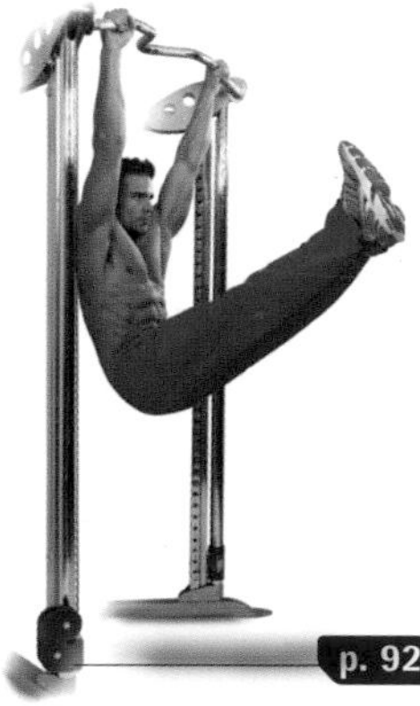

p. 46

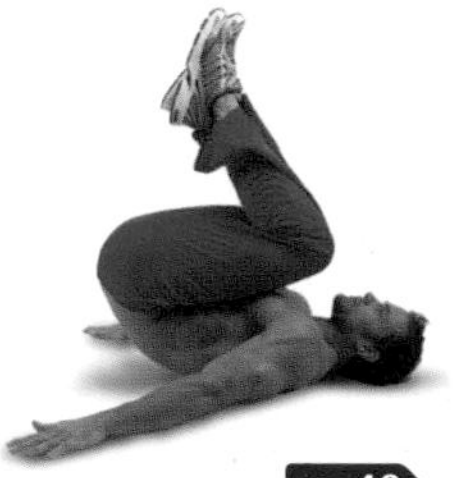

p. 92

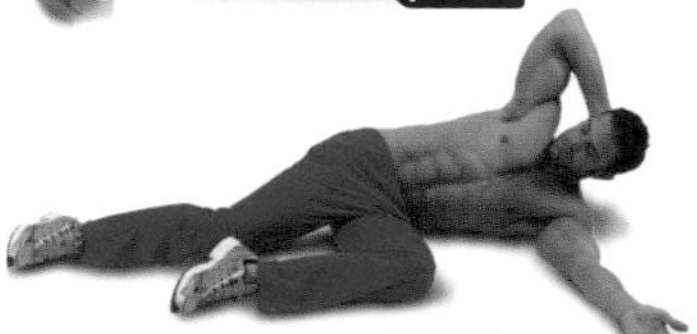

p. 56

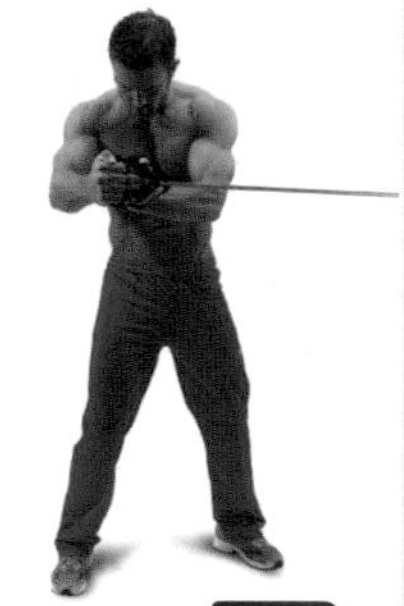

p. 112

WORKOUT 2

● **Double crunch with weight on the torso** — p. 44

12 to 8 repetitions; at fatigue, put down the
weight so you can immediately combine with

● **Classic crunch** — p. 40

Do the maximum number of repetitions:
5 sets with 1 minute of rest between sets.

● **Twisting crunch** — p. 54

4 sets of 40 to 25 repetitions with
no rest between the right and left sides.

● **Cable twist** — p. 112

A set to the right and then a set to the left
with no rest between the two:
4 sets of 50 to 30 repetitions.

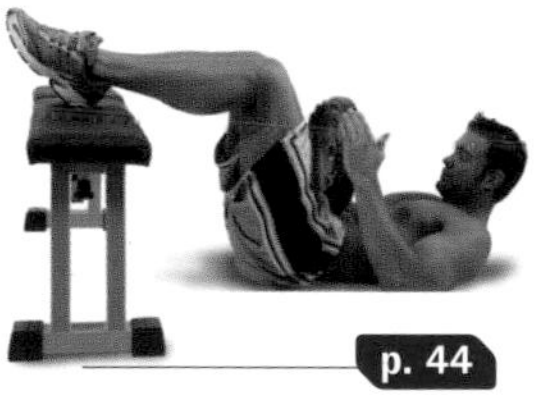

WORKOUT 3: Repeat the cycle.

p. 44

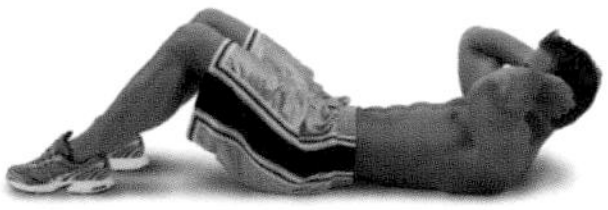

p. 40

p. 54

p. 112

SIX-PACK PROGRAMS

AT-HOME PROGRAMS Using Accessories

Swiss Ball Programs

Beginning Program

Do at least 2 times per week

● **Swiss ball crunch**   p. 104
3 sets of 20 to 15 repetitions with
30 seconds of rest between sets.
Spend this rest time on your back doing a

● **Relaxation stretch on a stability ball**   p. 71

● **Swiss ball crunch with side twist**   p. 105
2 sets of 15 to 12 repetitions.
Do all twists to the right
before beginning a set to the left.
Do not rest between the right and left sides.

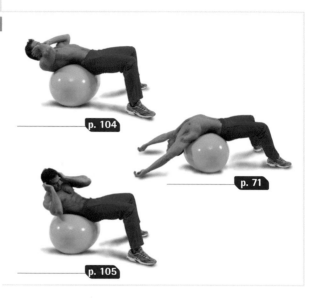

Advanced Program

Do at least 3 times per week
5 NONSTOP CIRCUITS

A circuit consists of combining these two exercises
with no rest:

● **Swiss ball crunch**   p. 104
20 to 15 repetitions until fatigue;
end the set with **crunches on the floor**.

● **Swiss ball crunch with side twist**   p. 105
15 to 12 repetitions to the right.
When you reach fatigue, end the set

● **on the floor**   p. 54
then move to the left side.

After 5 circuits, end your workout with

● **Relaxation stretch on a stability ball**   p. 71

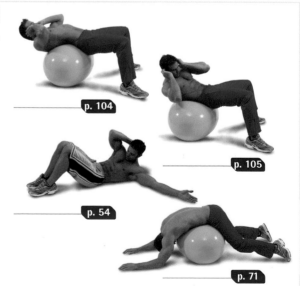

Ab Coaster Programs

Beginning Program

Do at least 2 times per week

● Straight Ab Coaster   p. 110
   3 sets of 12 to 8 repetitions with
   30 seconds of rest between sets.

● Twisting Ab Coaster   p. 111
   2 sets of 10 to 8 repetitions with
   no rest between the right and left sides.

p. 110   p. 111

Advanced Program

Do at least 3 times per week

● Straight Ab Coaster   p. 110
   12 to 8 repetitions; at fatigue,
   combine immediately with

● Lying leg raise   p. 46
   Do the maximum number of repetitions:
   5 sets with 45 seconds of rest between sets.

● Twisting Ab Coaster   p. 111
   10 to 8 repetitions; at fatigue,
   combine immediately with

● Side crunch   p. 56
   Do the maximum number of repetitions:
   3 sets with 15 seconds of rest once you
   have done the right and left sides.

p. 110   p. 46

p. 111   p. 56

Rocking Machine Programs

Beginning Program

Do at least 2 times per week

● Rocking machine crunch   p. 106
   5 sets of 25 to 15 repetitions with
   20 seconds of rest between sets.

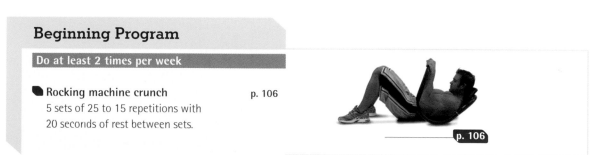

p. 106

SIX-PACK PROGRAMS

Advanced Program

Do at least 4 times per week

● **Rocking machine crunch** p. 106
5 sets of 35 to 25 repetitions with
15 seconds of rest between sets.

● **Rocking machine crunch on the side** p. 106
3 sets of 20 to 15 repetitions with
no rest between the right and left sides.

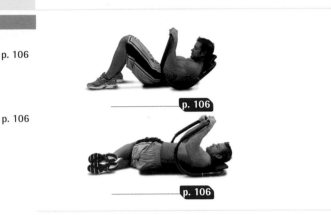

PROGRAMS Using Equipment in a Gym

Beginning Program

Do at least 2 times per week

● **Machine crunch** p. 103
5 sets of 25 to 8 repetitions with
30 seconds of rest between sets.
Increase the weight with every set.

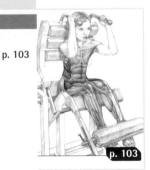

Advanced Program

Do at least 3 times per week

● **Hanging leg raise** p. 90
4 sets of 12 to 8 repetitions with
45 seconds of rest between sets.

● **Machine crunch** p. 103
3 sets of 15 to 8 repetitions with
30 seconds of rest between sets.
Increase the weight with every set.

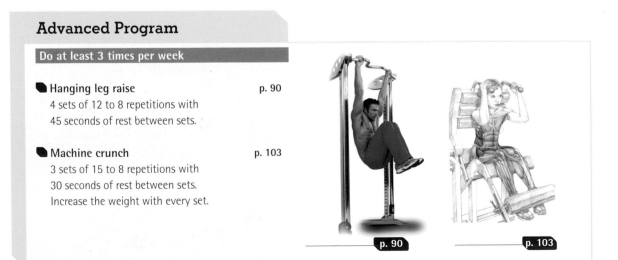

PROGRAMS to Reduce Belly Fat

These programs are for people who want to chisel abdominal muscles, lose belly fat, and slim down the waist. This workout can be done in the morning or the evening (or at both times) to improve blood circulation in the abdominal area throughout the day. The rhythm of the repetitions will be a little faster than normal but always without any abrupt movements, particularly in the low back.

Beginning Program

Do at least 3 times per week

3 NONSTOP CIRCUITS

of these combined exercises, done without rest breaks:

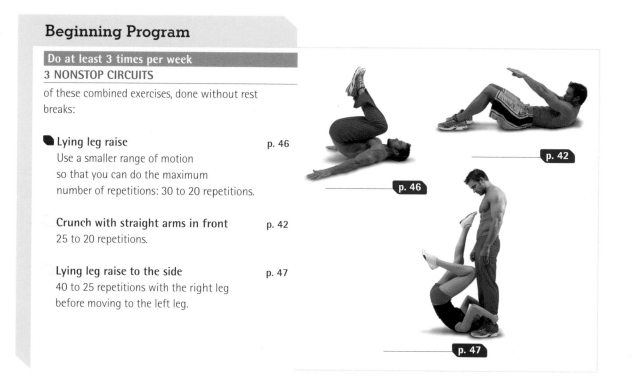

● **Lying leg raise**   p. 46
Use a smaller range of motion so that you can do the maximum number of repetitions: 30 to 20 repetitions.

Crunch with straight arms in front   p. 42
25 to 20 repetitions.

Lying leg raise to the side   p. 47
40 to 25 repetitions with the right leg before moving to the left leg.

Advanced Program

Do at least 4 times per week

4 NONSTOP CIRCUITS

Seated leg raise   p. 50
30 to 25 repetitions.

Crunch with hands on shoulders   p. 42
25 to 20 repetitions.

● **Side crunch**   p. 56
40 to 20 repetitions on the right side before moving to the left side.

SIX-PACK PROGRAMS

Very Advanced Program

Do at least 5 times per week
4 OR 5 NONSTOP CIRCUITS

Double crunch p. 79
20 to 15 repetitions.

Seated leg raise p. 50
35 to 20 repetitions.

Twisting crunch p. 54
40 to 20 repetitions on the right side
before moving to the left side.

Side crunch p. 56
30 to 15 repetitions on the right side
before moving to the left side.

PROGRAMS to Reduce Love Handles

Beginning Program

Do at least 3 times per week
3 NONSTOP CIRCUITS OF 30 TO 25 REPETITIONS

Twisting crunch p. 54
Once you have done the right side,
move on to the left side.

Cable twist p. 112
A set to the right and then a set to the left.

Advanced Program

Do at least 4 times per week
5 NONSTOP CIRCUITS OF 50 TO 30 REPETITIONS

Lying twist p. 98
A set to the right and then a set to the left.

Cable twist p. 112
A set to the right and then a set to the left.

Twisting crunch p. 54
A set to the right and then a set to the left.

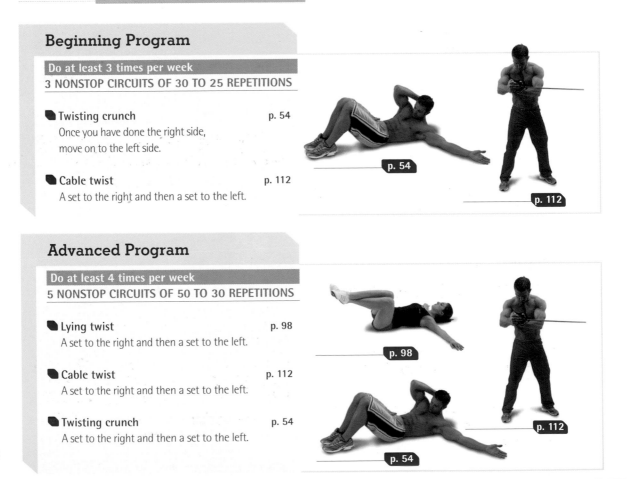

PROGRAMS to Highlight Apollo's Belt

Beginning Program

Do at least 2 times per week

● Twisting crunch   p. 54
Do small twists at the beginning of the exercise:
5 sets of 30 to 15 repetitions.
Do a set to the right and then a set to the left,
with no rest between the 2 sets.

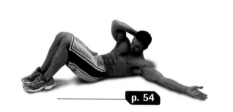

Advanced Program

Do at least 3 times per week

● Twisting crunch   p. 54
Do small twists at the beginning
of the exercise:
5 sets of 50 to 25 repetitions with no rest
between the right and left sides.

● Cable twist   p. 112
A set to the right and then a set
to the left with no rest between the sets:
3 sets of 30 to 15 repetitions.

PROGRAMS FOR WELL-BEING

PROGRAMS for Cardiovascular Health

Beginning Program

Do at least 2 times per week
Do the following circuit for 5 to 10 minutes.

● Lying leg raise   p. 46
Use a decreased range of motion so that you
can do the maximum number of repetitions:
30 to 25 repetitions.

● Crunch with straight arms in front   p. 42
So that you can do the maximum number
of repetitions: 25 to 20 repetitions.

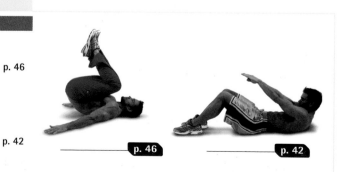

PROGRAMS FOR WELL-BEING

Advanced Program

Do at least 3 times per week

Do this circuit for 15 minutes.

● **Crunch with hands on shoulders**   p. 42
25 to 15 repetitions.

● **Seated leg raise**   p. 50
35 to 20 repetitions.

● **Side crunch**   p. 56
30 to 15 repetitions on the right side,
then immediately start the left side.

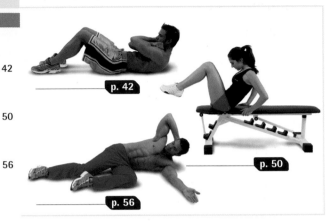

Very Advanced Program

Do at least 3 times per week

Do this circuit for 20 minutes.

● **Seated leg raise**   p. 50
With straight legs and then bent legs:
35 to 20 repetitions.

● **Double crunch**   p. 79
20 to 15 repetitions.

● **Twisting crunch**   p. 54
40 to 20 repetitions on the right side,
then immediately start the left side.

PROGRAMS to Relax Your Back Before Sleep

No Equipment Required

Beginning Program

Do this every night

● **Crunch**   p. 40
Do very slowly, with a small range of motion:
3 sets until your abdominal muscles are tired, with
30 seconds of rest between sets. These 30 seconds of
rest between crunches are devoted to the following:

● **Lying twist**   p. 98

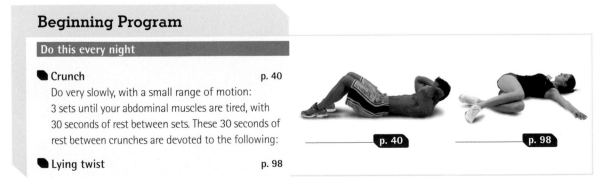

With Equipment

Beginning Program

Do this every night

🔴 **Crunch**   p. 40
Do very slowly, with a small range of motion:
2 sets until your abdominal muscles are tired, with
30 seconds of rest between sets. These 30 seconds of
rest between crunches are devoted to the following:

🔴 **Relaxation stretch on a stability ball**   p. 71

🔴 **Hanging from a pull-up bar**   p. 72
Relax your back for 30 seconds to 1 minute
by hanging from a pull-up bar
(support yourself intermittently
with your feet to relax your hands).

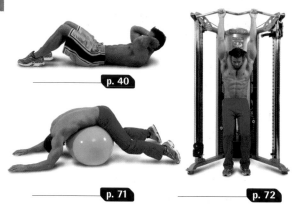

Advanced Program

Do this every night

🔴 **Crunch**   p. 40
Do very slowly, with a small range of motion:
2 sets until your abdominal muscles are tired,
with 1 minute of rest between sets:
• The first 30 seconds of rest between crunches
are spent doing

🔴 **Relaxation stretch on a stability ball**   p. 71
• The last 30 seconds of rest are spent doing

🔴 **Lying twist**   p. 98

🔴 **Hanging from a pull-up bar**   p. 72
Relax your back for 30 seconds to 1 minute
by hanging from a pull-up bar
(support yourself intermittently with
your feet to relax your hands).

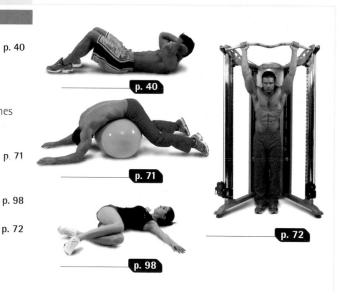

PROGRAMS FOR WELL-BEING

PROGRAMS to Help Protect Your Lumbar Spine

Beginning Program

Do at least 3 times per week

● **Crunch**   p. 40
Do very slowly, with a small range of motion:
2 sets of 20 to 15 repetitions with
30 to 45 seconds of rest in between sets.
These 30 seconds of rest between crunches
are spent stretching your hip flexors by doing

● **Lunge**   p. 68
Hold the stretch in each thigh for at least
15 seconds without arching your back.

● **Static stability, back against wall**   p. 58
4 sets of at least 10 seconds each with
30 seconds of rest between sets.
Spend this rest time

● **Hanging from a pull-up bar**   p. 72
Relax your back for 15 to 30 seconds
while you hang suspended.

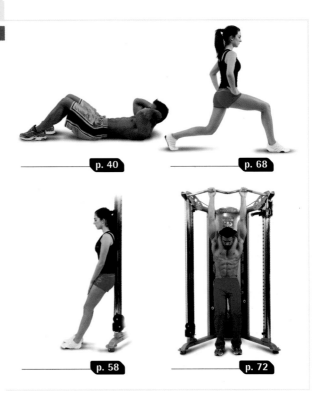

p. 40   p. 68

p. 58   p. 72

Advanced Program

Do at least 4 times per week

● **Double crunch**   p. 79
3 sets of 25 to 12 repetitions with 30 to 45 seconds
of rest between sets. Spend these 30 seconds of rest
stretching your hip flexors by doing

● **Lunge**   p. 68
Hold the stretch in each thigh for at least
20 seconds without arching your back.

● **Twisting crunch**   p. 54
Do very slowly, with a small range of motion:
3 sets of 15 to 12 repetitions with
30 to 45 seconds of rest. Spend these
30 seconds stretching your lumbar spine by

● **Hanging from a pull-up bar**   p. 72
Support yourself intermittently with
your feet to relax your hands.

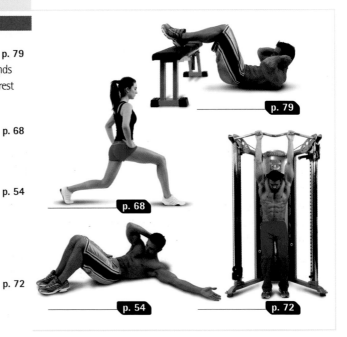

p. 79

p. 68

p. 54   p. 72

PROGRAMS to Help With Bloating and Other Digestive Problems

Beginning Program

Do at least 4 times per week

● **Double crunch**   p. 79
3 sets of 15 to 12 repetitions with
30 to 45 seconds of rest between sets.
Spend this rest time doing

● **Static stability, back against wall**   p. 58
2 sets of at least 10 seconds each.

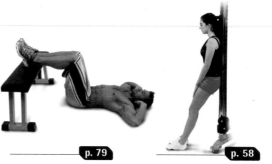

p. 79   p. 58

Advanced Program

Do at least 5 times per week

● **Lying leg raise**   p. 46
3 sets of 15 to 12 repetitions with
30 to 45 seconds of rest between sets.
Spend this rest time doing

● **Static stability, back against wall**   p. 58
3 sets of at least 15 seconds each.

● **Double crunch**   p. 79
3 sets of 15 to 12 repetitions with
30 to 45 seconds of rest between sets.
Spend this rest time doing

● **Diaphragm contraction**   p. 64
5 repetitions of at least 10 seconds each.

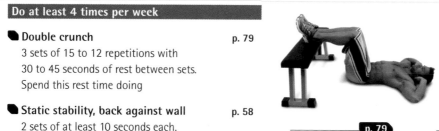

p. 46   p. 58

p. 79   p. 64

SPORT-SPECIFIC CORE PROGRAMS

Complexity of Athletic Programs

Strength training programs for sports are the most difficult to develop because they must be tailored to your individual needs. To do this well, you need to determine the following:

- Which core muscles are most often used in your sport
- Which qualities are required of those muscles (such as power, strength, or endurance).

These multiple demands require the development of very unique programs depending on the primary athletic discipline.

Circuit Training or Sets?

Is it better to work your core in a circuit or by doing regular sets? Every athlete has to answer this question individually.

Scientific studies provide interesting elements that we can analyze. Imagine two groups of beginning tennis players:

- The first group practices forehand shots repetitively. Once they have mastered that, they learn backhand shots the same way. This is similar to a workout using sets.
- The second group has to alternate forehand and backhand shots randomly. This is similar to a workout using circuits.

SPORT-SPECIFIC CORE PROGRAMS

At the end of the tennis lesson, both groups had done exactly the same number of forehand and backhand shots. Performance tests were done just after the lesson and repeated 10 days later.

Immediately after the lesson, the players who learned the shots in a repetitive fashion had made the most progress. But after 10 days, the players who trained with random shots in a circuit had improved their game the most.

These results demonstrate two things:

1. When you need to learn a new exercise quickly, it is better to repeat it in sets. If you're new to strength training, you should avoid circuits in the first few weeks of exercising so that you can learn how to perform core exercises properly. Doing circuits would just complicate the learning process for an exercise that is already difficult to master.

2. But very quickly, when your goal is to make your muscles as functional as possible, you will find that it is often better to work your core using circuits.

Conclusion

If your goal is to get nice-looking abs, it is not helpful to work out in circuits (except to eliminate fat). Circuits require adaptations from the cerebral and nervous systems that will not help improve your muscle tone. The only reason to do circuits in this case is if you need to save time.

To get functional core muscles, the complexity of your strength training routine should approach what you encounter on the field or court. This way, the workout will prepare your core muscles, endurance, and nervous system for the technical difficulties encountered in your sport.

PHENOMENON OF TRANSFER

When you do strength training to improve performance, it is clear that there is a transfer between the increase in strength achieved in the gym and the increase in your athletic prowess on the field. For a beginner, this transfer happens pretty well. But the more advanced you are in your sport, the more problematic this transfer becomes.

To ensure an optimal transfer, your strength training routine should be as close as possible to what you do in your sport. This is why it is critical that you adjust workout programs to suit your own needs.

PHASE 1: Basic Muscle Conditioning

You should follow the phase 1 program for a few weeks so that you can learn to correctly master the most common exercises. When you feel comfortable, you can move on to circuit training (phase 2).

Basic Conditioning Program for Multiple Sports

Do this 2 or 3 times per week

Rest for 30 seconds between sets.

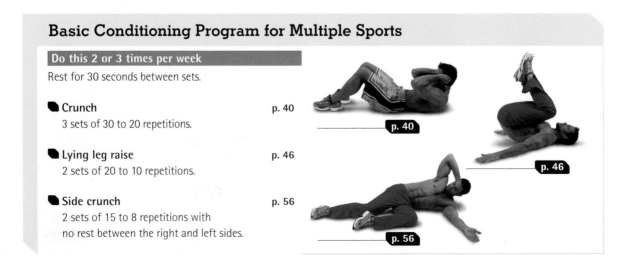

● **Crunch**   p. 40
3 sets of 30 to 20 repetitions.

● **Lying leg raise**   p. 46
2 sets of 20 to 10 repetitions.

● **Side crunch**   p. 56
2 sets of 15 to 8 repetitions with
no rest between the right and left sides.

PHASE 2: Circuit Training

After doing the phase 1 program for at least 2 weeks, it is time to begin circuit training.

Basic Conditioning Circuit for Multiple Sports

Do this 2 or 3 times per week

2 OR 3 CIRCUITS

(with no rest) including the following:

- 25 to 8 repetitions for strength sports
- 50 to 25 repetitions for sports requiring a good amount of endurance

🔲 Double crunch   p. 79

🔲 Seated leg raise   p. 50

🔲 Lying twist   p. 98

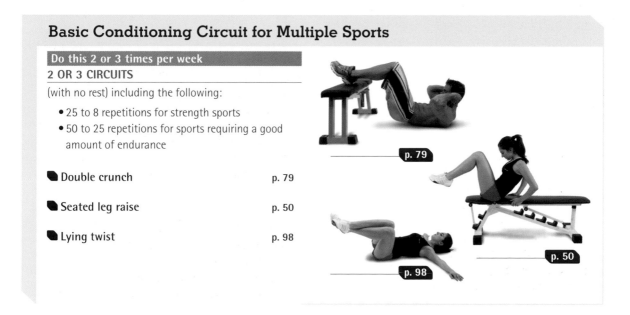

p. 79

p. 50

p. 98

PHASE 3: Improving Overall Physical Qualities

Programs for Torso Rotation

There are many sports in which the movement is initiated by torso rotation. For example, the power of a golfer's swing is acquired during the windup when he brings his club as high as possible before lowering it to hit the ball. A boxer's punch is initiated by rotating the torso to the back as a kind of windup. So it is important to strengthen the muscles responsible for this rotation so that you can

- gain power,
- increase endurance, and
- prevent injuries that are very common in this relatively fragile area of the body.

Beginning Program to Strengthen the Muscles Used for Torso Rotation

Do this 2 or 3 times per week

2 TO 4 CIRCUITS OF 50 TO 25 REPETITIONS

A circuit consists of the following exercises with no rest:

🔲 Twisting crunch   p. 54

🔲 Cable twist   p. 112

p. 54

p. 112

SPORT-SPECIFIC CORE PROGRAMS

Advanced Program to Strengthen the Muscles Used for Torso Rotation

Do this 4 times per week
3 TO 6 CIRCUITS OF 40 TO 15 REPETITIONS

● Hanging leg raise to the side   p. 96

● Cable twist   p. 112

● Twisting crunch   p. 54

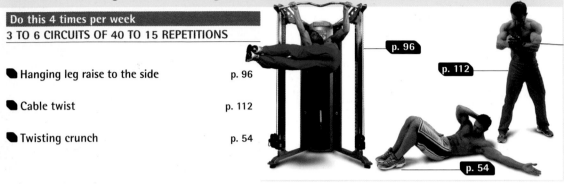

p. 96

p. 112

p. 54

Beginning Program for Respiratory Endurance

3 NONSTOP CIRCUITS

● Lying leg raise   p. 46
20 to 12 repetitions with 45 seconds of rest
between sets.
Spend this rest time doing

● Diaphragm contraction   p. 64
30 to 20 contractions.

● Crunch   p. 40
3 sets of 15 to 12 repetitions with
30 to 45 seconds of rest between sets.
Spend this rest time doing

● Lying rib cage expansion with a weight   p. 63
30 to 20 repetitions.

p. 46

p. 64

p. 40

p. 63

Advanced Program for Respiratory Endurance

5 NONSTOP CIRCUITS

● Seated leg raise   p. 50
15 to 12 repetitions with 30 seconds
of rest between sets.
Spend this rest time doing

● Diaphragm contraction   p. 64
40 to 30 contractions.

● Double crunch   p. 79
15 to 12 repetitions with 30 seconds
of rest between sets.
Spend this rest time doing

● Lying rib cage expansion with a weight   p. 63
50 to 30 repetitions.

p. 50

p. 64

p. 79

p. 63

PHASE 4: Sport-Specific Training

After one or two months of regular workouts, it is time to focus more specifically on the core muscles involved in your particular sport. In fact, every sport uses the muscles in the abdominal wall in a unique way. You should also be able to modify the sample programs and replace some of the exercises with ones that are particularly beneficial to you. We have included over 20 of the most common sports to help you find the program that works best for you.

Soccer

▶ The goal of this program is to strengthen the rotator muscles in the torso and the hip flexors while protecting the back.

Do this 2 or 3 times per week
2 TO 5 CIRCUITS OF 50 TO 20 REPETITIONS

Sit-up	p. 80
Seated leg raise	p. 50
Twisting crunch	p. 54
Static stability, back against wall For 30 seconds to 1 minute.	p. 58

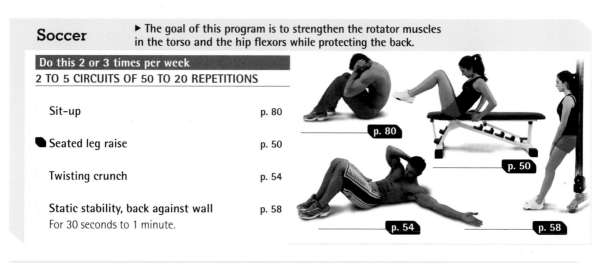

Cycling • Track Cycling

▶ The goal of this program is to strengthen the hip flexors and protect the back.

Do this 2 to 4 times per week
3 TO 5 CIRCUITS OF 12 TO 8 REPETITIONS

Sit-up	p. 80
Static stability, back against wall For 30 seconds to 1 minute.	p. 58
Seated leg raise	p. 50
Plank For 20 seconds to 1 minute.	p. 60

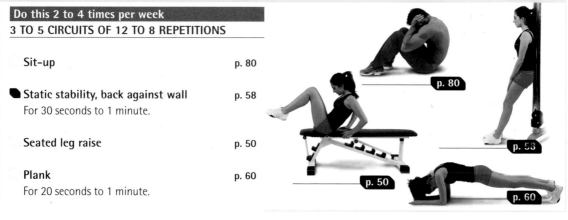

Cycling • Road Cycling

▶ The goal of this program is to strengthen the hip flexors and the muscles used for breathing while protecting the back.

Do this 1 to 3 times per week
2 TO 4 CIRCUITS OF 50 TO 30 REPETITIONS

Sit-up	p. 80
Lying rib cage expansion with a weight	p. 63
Seated leg raise	p. 50
Plank For 20 seconds to 1 minute.	p. 60

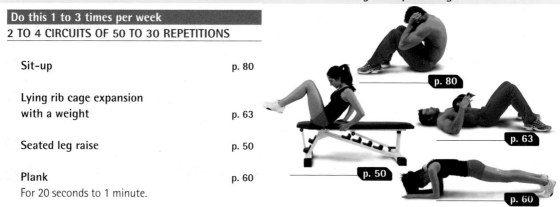

137

SPORT-SPECIFIC CORE PROGRAMS

Racket Sports

▶ The goal of this program is to strengthen the rotator muscles in the torso and the hip flexors.

Do this 1 or 2 times per week
2 TO 4 CIRCUITS OF 50 TO 12 REPETITIONS

- Sit-up   p. 80
- Cable twist   p. 112
- Side crunch   p. 56
- Twisting crunch   p. 54

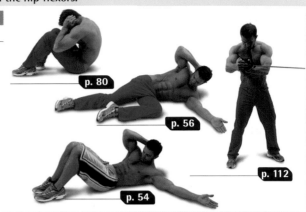

Rugby, American Football
and Team Contact Sports

▶ The goal of this program is to strengthen the rotator muscles in the torso and the hip flexors while increasing abdominal strength.

Do this 2 or 3 times per week
2 TO 5 CIRCUITS OF 30 TO 8 REPETITIONS

- Seated leg raise   p. 50
- Plank   p. 60
  For 20 seconds to 1 minute.
- Sit-up   p. 80
- Cable twist   p. 112

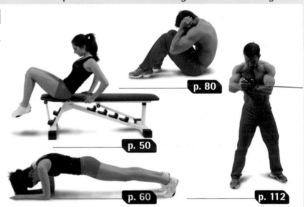

Basketball, Volleyball, Handball

▶ The goal of this program is to strengthen the rotator muscles in the torso, upper abs, and hip flexors.

Do this 2 or 3 times per week
2 TO 4 CIRCUITS OF 30 TO 12 REPETITIONS

- Sit-up while throwing a medicine ball   p. 84
- Cable twist   p. 112
- Twisting crunch   p. 54

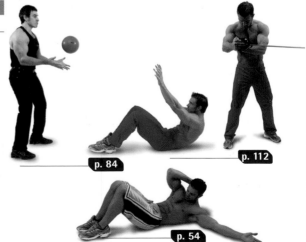

Downhill Skiing

▶ The goal of this program is to strengthen the abdominal muscles and protect the back.

Do this 2 or 3 times per week
4 TO 6 CIRCUITS

Plank   p. 60
For 20 seconds to 1 minute.

Crunch   p. 40
30 to 12 repetitions.

Static stability, back against wall   p. 58
For 30 seconds to 1 minute.

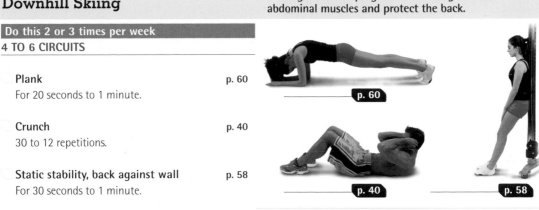

Cross-Country Skiing

▶ The goal of this program is to strengthen the hip flexors and the muscles used for breathing.

Do this 2 times per week
2 TO 4 CIRCUITS

Sit-up   p. 80
30 to 20 repetitions.

Lying rib cage expansion with a weight   p. 63
100 to 30 repetitions.

Plank   p. 60
For 20 seconds to 1 minute.

Diaphragm contraction   p. 64
100 to 30 repetitions.

Combat Sports

▶ The goal of this program is to strengthen the rotator muscles in the torso and the hip flexors while increasing abdominal strength.

Do this 2 or 3 times per week
4 TO 6 CIRCUITS OF 30 TO 8 REPETITIONS

Hanging leg raise   p. 90

Side plank   p. 60
For 15 seconds to 1 minute.

Sit-up while throwing a medicine ball   p. 84

Cable twist   p. 112

Twisting crunch   p. 54

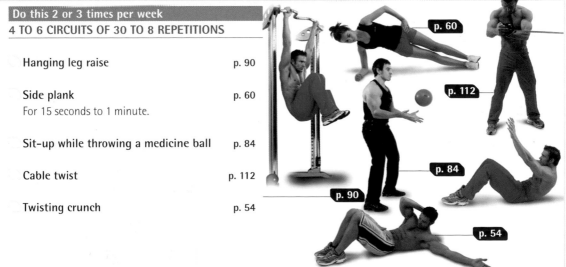

SPORT-SPECIFIC CORE PROGRAMS

Track and Field • Sprinting and Jumping

▶ The goal of this program is to strengthen the hip flexors and the obliques.

Do this 2 or 3 times per week

⬤ **Hanging leg raise**　　　　p. 90
4 to 6 sets of 8 to 1 repetitions with the maximum amount of weight.

⬤ **Twisting crunch**　　　　p. 54
4 to 6 sets of 12 to 8 repetitions with the maximum amount of weight.

⬤ **Sit-up**　　　　p. 80
2 sets of 10 to 8 repetitions with the maximum amount of weight.

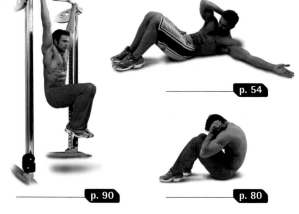

p. 54
p. 90
p. 80

Track and Field • Endurance Running

▶ The goal of this program is to strengthen the hip flexors and the muscles used for breathing.

Do this 1 to 3 times per week
2 TO 5 CIRCUITS

• 40 to 20 repetitions for events that are less than 5 minutes
• 100 to 50 repetitions for longer events

⬤ **Sit-up**　　　　p. 80

⬤ **Lying rib cage expansion with a weight**　　　　p. 63

⬤ **Seated leg raise**　　　　p. 50

⬤ **Diaphragm contraction**　　　　p. 64

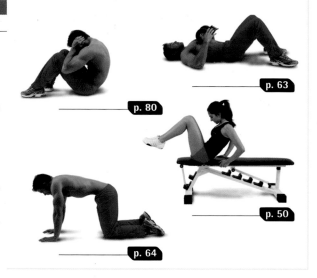

p. 63
p. 80
p. 50
p. 64

Track and Field · Shot Put

▶ The goal of this program is to strengthen the rotator muscles in the torso.

Do this 3 times per week

Twisting crunch p. 54
4 to 6 sets of 8 to 1 repetitions with the maximum amount of weight.

Side crunch p. 56
3 to 5 sets of 8 to 1 repetitions with the maximum amount of weight.

Swiss ball crunch p. 104
2 sets of 10 to 8 repetitions with the maximum amount of weight.

Cable twist p. 112
2 sets of 30 to 20 repetitions.

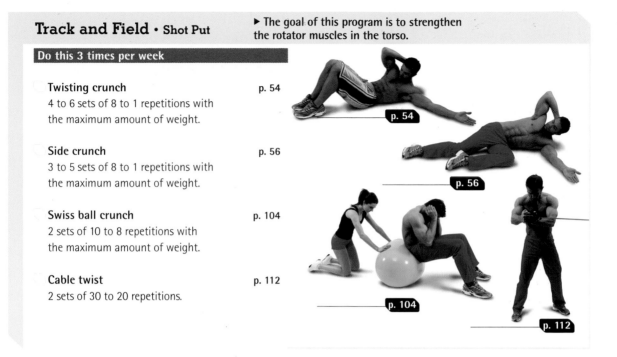

p. 54

p. 56

p. 104

p. 112

Swimming

▶ The goal of this program is to strengthen the rotator muscles in the torso and the muscles used for breathing.

Do this 2 to 4 times per week
4 TO 6 CIRCUITS OF 75 TO 25 REPETITIONS

Swiss ball crunch p. 104

Lying twist p. 98

Twisting Swiss ball crunch p. 105

Cable twist p. 112

p. 104

p. 105

p. 98

p. 112

Golf

▶ The goal of this program is to strengthen the rotator muscles in the torso and protect the back.

Do this 1 or 2 times per week
2 OR 3 CIRCUITS OF 20 TO 8 REPETITIONS

Cable twist p. 112

Twisting crunch p. 54

Crunch p. 40

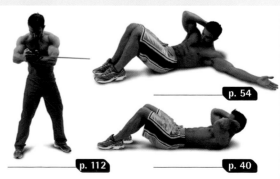

p. 54

p. 112

p. 40

SPORT-SPECIFIC CORE PROGRAMS

Ice Sports • Ice Skating, Hockey

▶ The goal of this program is to strengthen the rotator muscles in the torso and the hip flexors.

Do this 2 or 3 times per week
2 TO 5 CIRCUITS OF 40 TO 10 REPETITIONS

◗ Twisting crunch — p. 54

◗ Sit-up — p. 80

◗ Cable twist — p. 112

p. 54

p. 80

p. 112

Water Sports • Rowing

▶ The goal of this program is to strengthen the upper abdominal muscles and the muscles used for breathing while protecting the back.

Do this 2 to 4 times per week
2 TO 5 CIRCUITS OF 40 TO 20 REPETITIONS

◗ Sit-up — p. 80

◗ Lying rib cage expansion with a weight — p. 63

◗ Static stability, back against wall — p. 58
For 30 seconds to 1 minute.

◗ Diaphragm contraction — p. 64

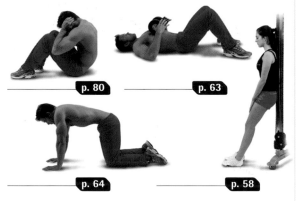

p. 80

p. 63

p. 64

p. 58

Water Sports • Kayak, Sailing

▶ The goal of this program is to strengthen the obliques and the upper abdominal muscles.

Do this 2 or 3 times per week
3 TO 5 CIRCUITS OF 50 TO 35 REPETITIONS

◗ Twisting crunch — p. 54

◗ Cable twist — p. 112

◗ Crunch — p. 40

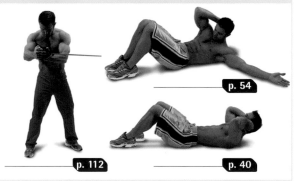

p. 54

p. 112

p. 40

Climbing

▶ The goal of this program is to strengthen the lower abdominal muscles, hip flexors, and obliques.

Do this 2 or 3 times per week

4 TO 6 CIRCUITS OF 50 TO 12 REPETITIONS

Hanging leg raise   p. 90

Twisting crunch   p. 54

Sit-up   p. 80

Plank   p. 60
For 20 seconds to 1 minute.

p. 54

p. 80

p. 90

p. 60

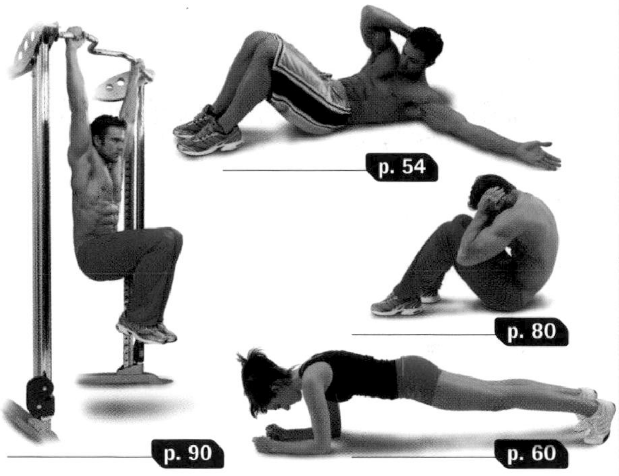

Motor Sports

▶ The goal of this program is to strengthen the abdominal muscles and protect the spine.

Do this 1 or 2 times per week

4 OR 5 CIRCUITS

Plank   p. 60
For 20 seconds to 1 minute.

Static stability, back against wall   p. 58
For 30 seconds to 1 minute.

Side plank   p. 60
For 10 to 20 seconds each side.

Static stability, back against wall   p. 58
For 30 seconds to 1 minute.

p. 60

p. 60

p. 58

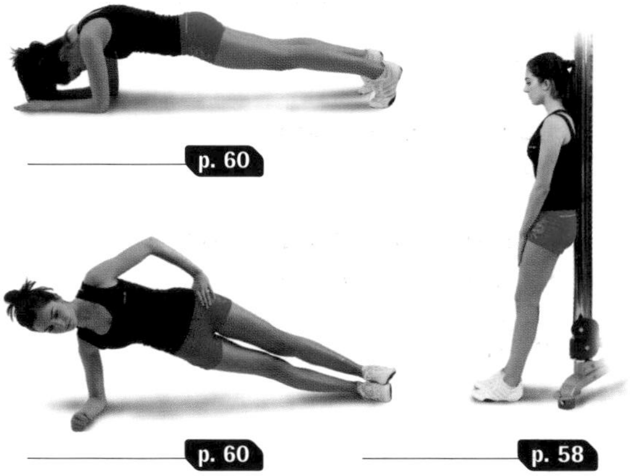

Exercise Index